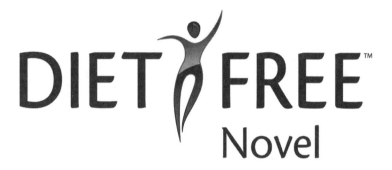

DIET FREE™

Novel

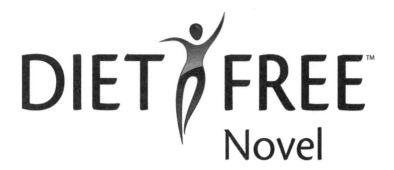

# DIET FREE™
## Novel

### The Inspiring Story Of
### The Eight Habits That Will Change Your Life

*Water*
*with*
*Lemon*

## Zonya Foco, RD and Stephen Moss

ISBN 10: 1-890926-10-8
ISBN 13: 978-1-890926-10-6

Library of Congress Control Number: 2006905851

PRINTED IN THE UNITED STATES OF AMERICA

Published by ZHI Publishing

*Water with Lemon* by ZHI Publishing (2006) is a fully revised and updated edition that replaces Stephen Moss's previously published *Lose Weight with The Power of One* published by Stephen Moss, August 2003.

*Water with Lemon* is available at special discounts for bulk purchase. Special editions can also be created to specification. For details, contact the Director of Marketing at ZHI Publishing.

Direct reproduction requests and any questions to the authors at:
    ZHI Publishing
    7134 Donegal Dr.
    Onsted, MI 49265
    Phone: 517-467-6995
    Fax: 517-467-7468
    E-mail: contact@Zonya.com
    Website: www.Zonya.com

To order additional copies, visit www.Zonya.com or call toll-free 888-884-5326.

Photos of Zonya: Tom Nakielski, Lights On Studio, Lansing, Michigan
Photos of Stephen: Richard Mayoff, Montreal, Canada
Book Cover Design: Kaplan Studio, Cary, North Carolina

Manufactured in the United States

This book is intended as a reference to healthy eating and exercise. It is not intended as a substitute for any treatment prescribed by your doctor. It is recommended that everyone receive regular checkups from a medical doctor and inquire specifically about nutrition and exercise recommendations. If you suspect that you have a medical problem, by all means, see your doctor.

# Foreword

Like many physicians, my time is limited. So when I was asked to read *Water with Lemon,* I hesitated. However, after reading just the first few pages, I found that I couldn't put the book down—and read it in its entirety in a single day.

As the Chief Medical Officer for Health Alliance Plan (HAP), one of Michigan's largest health plans, serving over 525,000 members, I am thrilled to recommend this simple yet profoundly inspiring story not only to HAP members, but to *everyone.* Whether overweight or not, managing high cholesterol, high blood pressure or diabetes, or simply seeking to improve your health, this book provides you with a realistic nutritional blueprint for health.

Adopting the habits presented in this book does work. In fact, more than 6,000 members of the HAP Weight Wise℠ Program have already begun experiencing their practical and powerful health and weight-loss benefits. And you can, too.

Read *Water with Lemon* and read it again. It will change your life!

Yours in good health,

Mary Beth Bolton, MD, FACP
Senior Vice President and Chief Medical Officer
Health Alliance Plan of Michigan

# Introduction from Zonya

## Knowing and Doing are Two Different Things

I'd been a trim kid until my junior year in high school, when I packed on 20 pounds. As a cheerleader whose place was in the middle of the "human pyramid," I heard my fellow teammates say, loud and clear, "Go on a diet!"

I took the problem to my mom and told her I had to lose 20 pounds, and I had to lose it by Friday's game. Together we concocted our own crazy weight loss combination of fasting and liquids. Like so many others, we thought this would get the most weight off in the quickest time. Unknowingly, I was actually discovering the quickest way to *gain* weight!

I spent the next four years yo-yo dieting, ending each effort heavier than I had been before. That's why I dedicated myself to becoming a dietitian: so I could master weight control in a healthy and permanent way. There was only one problem. I graduated from college at my highest weight ever! In our food-obsessed world, I discovered that *knowing* and *doing* are two different things, even for me.

## In Search of the Weight Control Answer

For eight years, I developed and taught weight and cholesterol-management programs at St. Joseph Mercy Hospital in Ann Arbor, Michigan. Through my own struggles and successes, and those of my clients, the pieces of the "permanent" weight-loss puzzle began to reveal themselves. I left St. Joe's and wrote the best-selling *Lickety-Split Meals For Health Conscious People on the Go* (the kitchen countertop coach that clients asked for), and began a professional speaking career teaching people across the nation about the *Power of One Good Habit*.

While my audiences loved *Lickety-Split Meals,* they still wanted me to write a "diet" book.

I'd read hundreds of clinical studies and just about every diet book on the shelf. From Atkins to the Zone, I found tiny "grains of truth" buried beneath diet hype and false diet hope. That's when I began my quest to extract the truth, delete the hype and focus on a common-sense message that leaves the diet mentality behind. Why couldn't cumbersome number counting be replaced by a few simple habits that each of us could *easily* and *realistically* rely on for the rest of our lives?

That's how my Eight Healthy Eating Habits for Life were born. I began teaching these eight habits from my speaking platform and on my TV show. And the results were phenomenal! The habits worked, and worked permanently! Now it was time to put these life-changing habits into a weight-loss book.

## A Force To Be Reckoned With

That's when I met Stephen, and we discovered how my eight proven habits and innovative approach to nutrition could be partnered with his own weight-loss strategies and emotionally charged storytelling talents, creating a force to be reckoned with!

The truth was revealed and a new genre was born: America's first health novel on weight loss: *Water with Lemon!*

Enjoy! Zonya

P.S. If any of the meals that Fowler or Karen prepares sound good to you, you'll find these *Lickety-Split Meals'* recipes posted for you at www.Zonya.com!

# Introduction
# from Stephen

I grew up in a household where my parents and sister were overweight. But I was one of those irritating types who could eat as they please and never gain an ounce—until I turned thirty. Then it hit me, too.

Overnight my weight jumped up 30 pounds. I crash-dieted that weight off, patted myself on the back, then turned around and gained it back, plus a little more. And this became my pattern for years. I tried every diet out there: low-fat, low-calorie, low-carb, and the last-as-long-as-you-can starvation diets!

Finally, fed up with feeling like a failure each time my willpower gave out and I ate what I really craved, I decided to find the answer to the question, "How can I lose weight easily, and keep it off, *without dieting?*"

During the next 10 years I read everything I could find on fitness and nutrition, along the way becoming a Specialist in Weight Management, a Lifestyle and Weight Management Consultant, and a Certified Fitness Trainer. Fitness and nutrition became a passion. I also discovered that the answer to my question had been there all along, but it was so deeply buried within dry clinical studies that it had to be mined, brought out bit by bit like gold nuggets from a mile-deep shaft.

The solution to permanent weight loss turned out to have virtually nothing in common with the fad diets I'd been attempting. The real answer was a combination of simple steps filled with common sense that fit easily into my daily life. I applied what I discovered and began to lose weight; slowly, continuously and *easily*. Without dieting. Until I lost all I had to. And since then I've lived my life as someone fit and healthy. I'd found the answer for my wife and myself, and we were happy to go on with our lives.

The story might have ended there, but as friends and family began asking me to help them also get their weight under control, I started to realize that my passion for health could also fit well with my other life passion: writing novels. Because from the beginning of time, the *story* has always been the best way to impart information.

I realized the novel form would allow me to write not just the facts of weight management, but to also portray the emotional roller-coaster all overweight people ride during their weight-loss journey. It would allow me to do what I wanted most: instill a strong sense of motivation and inspiration into my readers.

I drafted my story and found my characters, honing each one until they played a distinct role in the teaching of weight management and health through nutrition. Then I joined forces with Zonya Foco, and together we combined our skills and energies into producing America's first health novel. *Water with Lemon* is the first weight-loss guide that not only teaches the reader *how* to lose weight without dieting, but also motivates him or her into *doing it*.

Stephen

*When we adopt one seemingly insignificant change into our everyday lives, the result, over time, can surpass all expectations.*

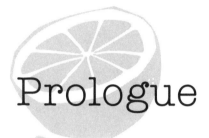

# Prologue

"I have been transformed," Karen wrote in her journal. "The Power of One Good Habit took me from fat to thin. Unhealthy to healthy. Self-conscious to self-confident."

She paused, reread what she'd just written, then underlined the words *thin, healthy* and *confident.*

From the back lawn came a shout, then laughter. Karen stood and stepped to the patio door to check on Gabe, her five-year-old, and was about to take her seat again when she caught sight of her reflection in the glass. All she had on was a pair of jeans and a T-shirt, but even after four years she was still thrilled to catch a glimpse of how she looked. And it had happened so easily, she thought. Without dieting! Simply by taking one small step, then another, and another.

That was all Fowler had asked of her. An incremental, consistent movement toward better health, toward losing weight. "Let the Power of One Good Habit slip into your world," he'd said. "Let each habit build on the next. Let the process be gradual, thoughtful. Let it become a *part* of your life, without intruding *into* your life."

He had talked about courage. Just the amount needed to learn what there was to learn. Then he'd placed his eight simple habits into a nest of creativity, promising, "That's all you'll ever need."

And he was right.

Karen smiled, remembering how she'd first resisted, then reluctantly agreed to listen to his words. Only that. Just listen.

And then the eight habits took hold.

"Thank you, Fowler," she whispered. "For showing me the way. For giving me back my life."

She returned to her desk and lifted the pen once again. But she didn't start writing. Instead she found her mind drifting back to how the transformation of her weight, and her life, had started.

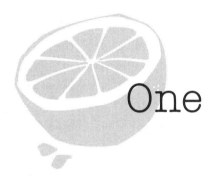

# One

The screen door slammed behind Karen. She hurried toward the dark woods at the back of the lawn, her six-month-old son crying in her arms. After a couple of steps she couldn't catch her breath. Halfway across the yard she slowed to a walk. And at the white oak that marked the beginning of the woods beyond her lawn's boundary, she stopped, pressed her shoulder against the tree, and fought for air.

The door behind her banged open and Gary stepped onto the porch, his belly hanging over the waistband of his red boxers.

Karen, struggling to calm Gabe, turned to face him, thinking, *This time he's going to have to beg to get me back! Promise to stop calling me names. I know I'm overweight, but that's not the cause of every problem we have!*

But Gary yelled, "You can say whatever you want, Karen! I don't care anymore. You're a fat cow and you make me sick!" He stormed back into the kitchen. The door slammed shut behind him.

Karen watched through the kitchen window as Gary took a few steps, seemed to change his mind, then lifted her purse from where she'd slung it over the back of a chair. He turned to face the window and, holding the purse high, yelled, "Running into the back wasn't a good idea, Karen, especially without this! 'Cause now I'm locking you out!" Then he slammed the storm door, slid the bolt and turned off the porch light, leaving the yard in blackness.

Karen was stunned. For a moment all she could do was stare at the door. Then she cursed softly, and clamped her jaws. Taking a deep breath to calm herself, she lowered her head to Gabe's. *Okay, Gary, you know I have no place to go. So you're waiting, expecting me to knock at the door, ask to be let in. Even apologize for standing up for myself! But that's not going to happen. I'll stay out all night before I give you that satisfaction!*

And with this, she turned toward the woods.

In the six weeks she'd lived here, she had never before gone beyond the perimeter of the lawn, had not yet found the time to see where her town-house community met the farmhouses and barns of a passing era.

*I don't have to go far,* she reasoned, her determination rising. *Just far enough so Gary will have to search for me when he starts to worry. Force him to bend a little. All I need is a place to sit, and I'll wait him out!*

The night was warm, the sky brilliant with stars. Karen, quickly winded again, kept her pace slow and let the rocking motion of her steps lull Gabe to sleep. She made her way through the woods until she came to a clearing where a split-rail fence lay forgotten. With Gabe in her lap, she sat next to one of the fence posts. Once more she struggled to regain her breath.

But now a familiar knot began to ache in her gut, a knot that had been tightening for years, clamping down with each pound gained. She sighed, hating the feeling, and realized

4

that after sixty extra pounds, the knot had finally twisted into hopelessness.

Then she heard a man's voice call out, "Courage!"

The word, a sudden shout in the night, startled her. It was as if her own spirit were urging her on, demanding strength. It came again: "Courage!" She held her breath, waited for more, then heard, the tone softer now, "Hey, boy. You see something? Is something there?"

A large dog bounded toward her from the trees. It stood barking on the other side of the fence until the voice commanded, "Courage! Get back here!"

The dog obeyed instantly, but the next moment Karen was blinded by a bright beam of light. She lifted her hand to shield her eyes. The light dropped to the ground. Gabe began to cry.

Karen blinked, tried to focus. The light, now held low, moved toward her. She could make out the outline of a man. He stopped about fifteen feet from where she sat, and once again lifted the light, though this time only until it illuminated the fence and Gabe. With her instincts on edge, Karen waited, thinking, *If there's even a hint of trouble, I'm running!*

But the man switched off his flashlight and gave a cautious greeting. The distance between them was too far for Karen to make out his features. He stepped closer, to just beyond arm's length from the fence and, dropping to one knee with the dog beside him, said, "Sorry about the light. We didn't know anyone was here. I hope Courage didn't scare you. He wouldn't harm a flea."

"It's okay," Karen answered. "We're fine."

The fence crossed Karen at chest height, creating a buffer. She rocked Gabe, quieting him again, and took a good look at the man.

He was lean. Lithe. Nearing or just past fifty, Karen guessed. His hair was thick and unruly and his cheeks were covered in a day's growth of stubble. He wore a pullover and a dark multi-pocketed vest, and jeans that were tucked into work boots. On his head was a lantern.

5

The man said, "My name's Fowler, and this is—"

"Courage," Karen said, the word sounding weak coming from her, not at all the way it had sounded when snapped out by the man.

Fowler grinned.

Karen smiled back. Then, realizing that if she could make out Fowler's features so clearly, he could do the same to hers, she immediately lowered her head.

It was the thickness of her face she'd grown ashamed of, the roll of her second chin, the swell of fat that had become her waist. She suddenly wished she'd found a cave to hide in and not this clearing, so no one would see she was wearing Gary's old Bulls sweatshirt because her shirts had again gotten too small, or that she wore sweatpants because the only pants or skirts she could get around her were those fitted with elastic waistbands.

"Courage and I were just out gardening," Fowler said.

"Gardening?" Karen again raised her eyes to Fowler's, looking for the joke in his expression, but saw none.

"It's what I do," Fowler said. "Garden. Often at night. Then I write about it in magazines." For a moment the only sound was Courage's breathing. Then Fowler continued, "Lacewing. Lacewing larvae. I was checking how they're doing on the hostas."

"Really," Karen replied, not sure what to make of this conversation.

"Yes. Lacewing larvae. It's a good insect. We buy them—gardeners, I mean—and put them where there're mites. I don't like chemicals. Never have. Don't like anything I can't pronounce."

Karen nodded, going along with what he said although she had no idea what it meant.

"I put a whole slew of them on my hostas," Fowler continued, more animated now, "and they've done an excellent job. Better than I expected. And I'm out now because I can see them more clearly at night, the plants and the bugs and what they've done, because of my lights, the intensity of my

6

lights. This one," he said, lifting his flashlight, "and this one too," he added, touching the lamp on his head. Then he removed it and held it out toward Karen, as though for her inspection. "This is the kind they use in mines. You know, down in the shafts. Keeps your hands free." He smiled broadly. "Works well here too. In my world."

"I would never have thought of that," Karen said. "It sounds like you've got it all figured out."

Courage pushed a wet nose beneath Fowler's chin and nudged his neck. "And Courage likes to come with me," Fowler continued, "to keep me company. Isn't that so, old boy?"

"He's a beauty," Karen said, stretching her arm out so the dog could sniff her hand. "Shepherd, right?"

"Shiloh Shepherd, the biggest, most affectionate shepherd there is. A really special breed."

Karen gave the black and gray dog a gentle rub behind the ears. She said, "We had a dog when I was growing up. For years she was my best friend." Then she added, "Oh, sorry, I'm forgetting my manners. I'm Karen, and this is Gabe. We're your neighbors. From over there, just past the trees. We've been sort of . . . locked out." She said nothing else, giving Fowler a brief, forced smile, and was grateful when he didn't ask for details.

Courage whined lightly and again nudged Fowler's neck. Fowler stroked the dog, saying, "You want to go back home, don't you?" Turning to Karen, he added, "His best friend's in the house, and he hates to leave her for very long." He hesitated. "Are you two going to be all right out here?"

"Oh, yes," Karen replied, trying to sound as if she meant it.

Fowler looked unconvinced. "The house is just a stone's throw from here," he said. "The least I can do is offer a locked-out neighbor a chair to sit in and a cup of tea."

Before Karen had a chance to respond, Fowler stood, propped the flashlight under his chin and, with a little grunt, lifted the old fence rail off its post and placed it aside, creating a doorway.

Then he held out his hand.

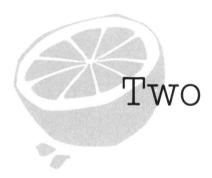

# TWO

Karen took Fowler's hand and stood, cringing at the thought that the first thing he was going to see was her size. The weight that had crept up when she hadn't been looking—weight that now ruled her life the way the black plague had ruled the Dark Ages.

Fowler gestured her to walk ahead of him on the narrow path, saying it was safer that way. "I'll be right behind you, almost at your side, so I can shine the light for both of us."

She stepped forward quickly, not wanting to catch his expression when he took in the thickness of her waist, the layers of fat on her thighs and buttocks. She held on tighter to Gabe, reassuring him with a gentle shushing sound that all would be well. Her thoughts though repeated a wish she had made too many times to count; that she could be thin the way others were thin. The way Fowler was thin. The way she had kept promising herself and Gary she'd become once again.

They walked through the trees for only a few minutes, with Courage leading the way and Fowler lighting the path so Karen could see where to step. He told her to watch out for a rock outcrop just ahead, and then to duck as they approached a low hanging branch. She could see little beyond Fowler's beam of light, but within a short distance the trees abruptly ended. Suddenly there was a park-like quality to the land, the perfume of a thousand flowers. She could sense a freshness here, one that was missing around the concrete rigidity of her town-house complex.

The path took an abrupt turn to the right and widened. Fowler stepped up beside her. Courage ran to a broad sweep of light coming from the back porch of a single-story farmhouse, the building squat, stone-solid, with a gable roof and overflowing window boxes.

*I've stepped back in time*, Karen thought, and with the thought came the odd realization that this place was only minutes from her kitchen window and she'd never known it was here. She turned to Fowler. "This is unbelievable!"

"It's out of the way now, sort of hidden, what with all the new developments," Fowler said, "but when I first moved here, there were only these old farmhouses."

Karen walked with Gabe onto the wide green-and-white porch and past a stout table flanked by heavy slatted chairs. Fowler reached out and opened the farmhouse's back door.

Courage rushed in first. Karen stepped into a large, wood-paneled cloakroom just in time to catch a last glimpse of the dog as he disappeared through a doorway at the end of a narrow hall. Fowler, placing his lamps on a wooden shelf and removing his vest, said, "If you'll excuse me for a moment, I'll just go tell my daughter we've got company." He hung his vest on a hook, stepped from the cloakroom and disappeared around the same corner Courage had taken.

Karen waited, still holding Gabe in her arms, her arms and back beginning to ache with the weight of him. She looked around the small room she was in, at the neat line of coats and raincoats hanging side by side, and at a collection of well-used terra-cotta pots stacked one into the other. She smiled at an old brass coat rack where an assortment of dog leashes shared equal space with a collection of garden clippers and worn gardening gloves.

Gabe squirmed in her arms. "I know," she whispered, "you should be in your crib now, not here." Her jaws tightened, the night's argument still fresh in her mind. *Can't you even try to understand, Gary? Not every problem we have needs to be turned into another fight over my weight! Why do you keep doing that?*

She heard the sound of voices, but they weren't loud enough for her to make out anything they were saying. For an instant she thought of just slipping out, then Fowler reappeared. Shaking his head, he said, "Sorry to be so long. Just a little family conference." He motioned toward a closed door set in the center of the hallway. He stepped to it, and opening it, said, "Please, the living room's in here. It's about time I showed you that chair I promised."

Karen stepped forward and through the doorway, ready to apologize for being here at all; but, taken by what she saw, she said instead, "Wow!"

The space she had just entered was large, lit by a series of matching wall lamps, their soft light reflecting off the worn, polished oak floor. One wall had four large wood-framed leaded windows, and another wall had two, with a bay window between them. What struck Karen first though were the plants; dozens of them, in all sizes and shapes and colors. They were hung from the ceiling on brass chains, and stood in pots on the floor. In front of the bay window, a pine table had begun to curve beneath the weight of a collection of flowering varieties.

In the center of the room, like a clearing on a tropical island, sat an overstuffed, cloth-covered easy chair, a low square wood table, and an old television with a DVD player on a stand. At the far end of the room stood a magnificent deep green tree in a terra-cotta pot that blocked all but a glimpse of what Karen thought must be the front door. Other plants, equally beautiful, filled the room.

Karen exclaimed when she saw them. "Your plants are beautiful!"

"Thank you. They're one of my passions," Fowler replied, saying more softly, "I guess that's obvious." Then he added, motioning to the largest plant in the room. "That's an aralia. I've had it forever. And this," he pointed to a green sprout in a tiny clay pot standing on the table next to the easy chair, "is my latest, sent to me from a reader in Arizona. I'm still studying it."

Along with the plant, the large cluttered table held textbooks and notepads, pencils and chalk, a wide glass bowl overflowing with fruit, and a pitcher of water with lemon slices and two glasses. Next to the pitcher was an old-fashioned magnifying glass and an open bag of potting soil.

Karen turned to the wall behind her, where a sofa, seemingly pushed out of the way, was stacked with magazines. But what really held her attention at this end of the room was an old-time schoolhouse blackboard mounted just a foot or so off the floor, entirely filling the wall. On the blackboard, in a small, neat script, was line after line of numbers and mathematical symbols.

"Have a seat," Fowler said, pointing to the easy chair. Then, as though noticing it for the first time, he stepped over to the coffee table and placed the bag of potting soil on the floor.

Karen first sat on the edge of the chair so she could adjust Gabe, who was now asleep. Then with a long sigh she sat fully into it. She looked up at Fowler and with a grateful smile said, "This is exactly what we needed." Then she gently covered Gabe's head with a corner of his blanket and leaned her head deeper into the chair.

For a moment Fowler stood awkwardly next to her, then, with another of his quick grins, said, "Guess I'd better clear a space for me, too." He stepped to the sofa and rearranged the magazines, then turning to Karen, said, "I promised you a tea, didn't I? I'll be right back."

Karen heard the clatter of cups and spoons from somewhere behind her. Again she heard Fowler speaking and assumed it was with his daughter. She sighed once more, feeling the tension leave her neck, and wondered if Gary had decided to go look for her yet, or if his stubborn streak still had him parked in front of the TV. She looked around the room again, soaking in its warmth, its endearing oddness. The blackboard told her that Fowler was not only an eccentric gardener, but also a scientist of sorts.

That he didn't have many visitors was clear.

She wondered too about the daughter, why she hadn't stepped in to say hello, been curious about a visitor. Karen let those thoughts drift away as she sank even deeper into the comfortable chair, realizing this was the first time she'd been able to relax in a long while. *Why can I do that here,* she wondered, *in just a matter of minutes, and yet never feel relaxed in my own home?*

Fowler returned with a tray in his hands. "I've been experimenting with herbal teas," he said. "At the moment, the one I like best is verbena." He poured the steaming water from a teapot into two cups. "It steeps quickly. In just a minute or two it reaches its full flavor."

Karen reached over Gabe and gratefully accepted the cup from Fowler. She first smelled the tea, nodding at its aroma, then took a sip and said, "This is excellent."

Fowler grinned. "I grow it myself, organically, and sundry it."

*Why am I not surprised to hear that?* Karen thought, taking a second sip. "I hope I'm not putting you or your daughter out."

But at that moment Fowler was looking past her, wearing a pleased, surprised expression. "Speaking of my daughter," he said, "here she is now!"

Karen tried to turn to greet her, but with the baby and

the cup of tea she couldn't turn quite far enough to see anything.

Fowler, still looking at his daughter, said, "It's all right . . . Why don't you join us?"

"I only wanted to see the baby." The voice was not loud, but strong, self-assured and strangely rough.

Karen set her cup down and looked behind her.

Fowler said, "Karen, this is Janice."

All Karen could see edging past the terra-cotta pot of the large tree was the front of an electric wheelchair. And feet. Tiny feet in white socks poking out from beneath a plaid wool blanket. Feet that were not much larger than Gabe's.

"Come and say hello," Fowler said. "I'm sure Karen would be happy to show you the baby."

Karen said, heartily, "Of course!" before her words stuck in her throat. The girl had her small hand around the black lever of the chair and had moved herself clear of the tree.

She was no more than three feet tall and sat in the chair at an awkward angle, shoulders slightly hunched. Her features were severely deformed, her skin color bruised shades of red. Karen was shocked. Courage, tail wagging, stood beside the wheelchair.

Karen heard Fowler say her name. She turned to him, eyes still wide.

"Janice has never seen a baby before," Fowler said calmly, his eyes holding Karen's.

"Except on TV," Janice added.

Karen, struggling to regain her composure, forced herself to look directly at the young woman. Somehow she found the words to say, "You can come closer. It's all right."

Janice inched her chair forward again, stopping it beside the TV. Karen lowered the blanket from Gabe's head and shoulders, revealing his blue pajamas. She watched as the girl's eyes lit up, thinking suddenly, *She's got the most beautiful eyes I've ever seen. So large and green.* She moved Gabe so that he faced Janice, and couldn't help but smile at Janice's expression of wonder.

"Can I get you a tea?" Fowler asked his daughter.

Janice hesitated visibly.

Karen glanced at Fowler and he gave her the slightest of nods. She turned to Janice. "Yes, please join us!"

Fowler stood. "I'll just get a cup. I'll be right back." He walked past his daughter, giving her shoulder a quick squeeze on his way out of the room.

In her odd gravelly voice, Janice asked, "What's the baby's name?"

"Gabe," Karen answered. "He just turned six months." Gabe's eyes were beginning to open. "Look, he's starting to wake up. Why don't you come a little closer, so you can really see him?"

Janice touched the lever on her wheelchair, stopping next to the easy chair. Still wearing a look of awe, she whispered, "He's beautiful."

"He is," Karen replied. "I mean, of course *I* think he is!" She laughed lightly.

Fowler returned with a cup for Janice. He filled it from the teapot, and, with a soft, "here you are," handed it to her. He was smiling. Beaming.

Karen watched as Janice took the cup from him. She sensed she was witnessing an important moment between them, but did not know why. Janice too was smiling, her large green eyes glowing.

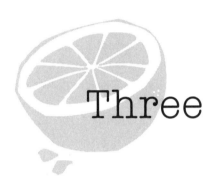

# Three

Fowler again took his seat, this time relaxing fully into it and crossing his legs.

Karen turned to him. He smiled at her but said nothing. Turning back to Janice, she said, "Would you like to touch Gabe?"

"Oh, yes!"

Karen said to Gabe, "Someone wants to say hello. Her name is Janice." She lifted Gabe, letting his blanket remain in her lap, and placed him in a seated position on the wide arm of the easy chair.

Janice reached out and touched one of Gabe's stockinged feet. Even for her small body, Janice's arms were too short, but Karen could see they were perfectly functional.

Janice said, "Hello, Gabe." Then, looking at Karen, she added, "He's so warm!"

"He is. Babies always seem that way. Put one of your fingers into his hand. See what happens."

Janice touched Gabe's palm with her forefinger and Gabe wrapped his fingers around it. Janice laughed.

Karen, still finding the sound unusually harsh, couldn't help laughing along with her. Fowler did the same, and Karen saw that his expression was now one of absolute pleasure.

"Is he hungry?" Janice asked Karen. Her hand was still firmly in Gabe's grip. Karen could see she was in no hurry to remove it.

"Not at all. He had a really good dinner about an hour ago. All he wants to do now is sleep. See, his eyes are beginning to close again."

"It's as though he's struggling to keep them open," Janice said.

For a few moments the three of them watched as Gabe's eyes slowly closed. Then Fowler said to Karen, "What about you? Are you hungry? Would you like something with your tea?"

Karen thought immediately, *That sounds good.* Then she gritted her teeth. *No! I'm not going to eat again until I've lost all my extra weight! Until there's no more reason for Gary to complain!*

Janice gave her a quick glance. "Is anything wrong?"

"No, no. I'm fine," Karen answered quickly.

"My father's a really good cook," Janice said.

"We'll let Karen decide that for herself," Fowler said, standing. "What'll it be? Something warm? Something cold? Something straight out of the garden? I have it all." He walked over to Janice and, standing beside her chair, stared down at Gabe, who was still holding on to Janice's finger.

"Something warm for me," Janice said, momentarily taking her eyes off Gabe to look at her father.

"There's one customer," Fowler grinned, getting a smile from Janice in return.

Karen said, "Nothing for me. Please, don't bother . . . "

"It's really no bother," Fowler said.

*Of course it's no bother,* Karen thought. *He can eat all he wants and enjoy it.* She hesitated for a moment before giving in to her hunger. "Okay, maybe just something small."

"Why don't we go into the kitchen, then?" Fowler said to Janice.

Janice nodded and, with obvious reluctance, pulled her finger from Gabe's grip.

Fowler said to Karen, "We're just going to move to the next room, but I should first tell you—"

"What he should tell you," Janice said, "is to brace yourself."

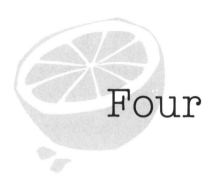

# Four

Karen wrapped Gabe in his blanket and stood. She followed Janice and Courage. Fowler, with their teas, the pitcher of water and the glasses all on the tray, was just behind her.

"This is the last thing I would have expected tonight," Karen said. "All I planned on doing was staying away from home for an hour or so, just until . . . " But the moment she stepped past the potted tree into the next room, the balance of her sentence was lost. "Oh, my! This is amazing!"

Janice said, "It's my father's restaurant."

"It *does* look like a restaurant, doesn't it?" Karen remarked, laughing lightly.

On one side of the room was a long wood table with another large bowl filled with fruit in the center, and beyond the table a glass-fronted, deli-style counter, softly underlit and curved at its ends to enclose the space behind it. The counter divided the room diagonally into two distinct parts, the eating and cooking areas.

"I always wanted my own restaurant—my kind of restaurant," Fowler said. "But I never needed to make a living from it. So I built it here, in my house." He stepped around the counter into the cooking area.

Karen, her smile a mix of delight and awe, continued to look around the room.

The walls were a combination of bricks and wooden beams, dotted with copper ornaments. Here too, along the walls, lush green plants hung from brass chains of varying lengths, creating a magnificent hanging garden. Flanking another large bay window were two enormous palm trees in terra-cotta pots. The window was framed by red-checked curtains.

Lined up neatly inside the serving counter were containers of all sizes, along with a carton of milk, a tray filled with assorted vegetables and a pot of peeled potatoes in water.

Fowler, standing behind the counter as though ready to take her order, said to Karen, "Come on in, and I'll give you the tour."

Karen shifted Gabe in her arms and stepped around the serving counter. Fowler started pointing out the kitchen's features. "Commercial stove, bakery oven, professional mixer and all the space I could ask for," he said. "Of course, no one needs all this in their house, but I like it."

"He's like a kid in here playing with his toys," Janice said.

"A chef's dream come true," Karen said, still astonished, as she looked at the chrome refrigerator and freezer, huge double sink, stainless-steel shelving and counter space, all of it gleaming.

"Why don't you have a seat?" Janice asked. "The baby must be getting heavy." She pointed to one of four high-backed chairs tucked into the long sides of the polished pine table. Karen nodded and, stepping out of the cooking area, gratefully took a seat, once again arranging Gabe in her lap.

At one end of the table was another collection of books and more papers and pencils.

Janice maneuvered her wheelchair to the head of the table next to Karen, saying, "This is where we spend most of our time." Courage, as though attached to Janice by an invisible leash, stayed at her side.

"If I had this kitchen, I'd never leave it," Karen said. Then, looking at the wall at the far end of the kitchen, she said with surprise, "What's that?"

On the wall was a pair of men's work trousers, size XXXL, spread wide and mounted in a frame, and on a shelf of its own, as though it were a trophy, a full bottle of Canadian whisky along with a package of cigarettes. Between those two items was an unlit, four-foot, blue neon sign that read, *The Power of One Good Habit.*

"The power of one good habit?" Karen repeated, turning to Fowler. "What does that mean?"

But Fowler was at the sink with his back to her, and Janice, her attention again fully on Gabe, said to Karen, "Look at his hands, they're little fists tucked under his chin."

Karen smiled at Janice. "He likes to sleep like that." She shifted Gabe slightly so she could continue to look around the room. She shook her head in wonder at the number and variety of plants, each one more exotic than the one before it, all of them arranged in a way that created the warmest, most inviting room she'd ever been in.

She turned to Fowler again, this time catching his eye, and quickly realized that from where he was standing he could clearly see her profile, see how Gabe rested on her stomach instead of her lap and how her thighs hung over the sides of the seat. Using the pretext of adjusting Gabe again, she let his blanket fall so that it hid most of her, too.

As she realized what she was doing, Karen lowered her head to the top of the baby's and sank into another overwhelming sense of hopelessness, aware yet again of just how much her weight controlled her life. She pictured what she looked like now—big round face, big body in an old sweat-shirt and sweatpants.

"Is there something we can do for Gabe?" Janice asked. "Does he need anything?"

At Janice's words, Fowler suddenly snapped his fingers and said, "I'll be right back." He stepped from the cooking area and hurried out a door at the far end of the kitchen.

Janice wore an expression that said this type of behavior should be expected from her father. "He's got an answer for every situation."

"I'm beginning to see that."

"I still get surprised," Janice continued, "but this time I can guess where he's going. To get my old cradle from the spare room."

Fowler quickly returned with a wooden cradle and a blanket. "This should do nicely," he said, putting the cradle on the floor between Karen's and Janice's chairs. He put in the blanket and then gave it a nudge so that it began to rock.

"It's beautiful," Karen said, admiring the rich, dark wood.

"We bought it just before Janice was born," Fowler said, holding out his hands for Gabe. Karen handed him the sleeping baby, and Fowler placed him gently into the cradle. He watched Gabe for a moment, then stepped behind the counter again.

Karen, leaning toward Janice, asked softly, "May I use your bathroom?"

"Of course," Janice said. "It's just outside there." She pointed to the door Fowler had used.

When Karen returned, she saw that Janice had turned her wheelchair so she could watch Gabe more easily. "He moves a lot when he sleeps," Janice remarked. Courage was stretched out on the floor beside Janice's chair. He thumped his tail as Karen took her seat.

On the table were three fresh teas and three glasses of water with lemon. Fowler was taking some cellophane-wrapped items from the freezer. He removed the wrappings and placed their contents in a glass dish, then covered the dish and put it into a microwave oven and set the timer. He took two more containers from the refrigerator. He uncovered the smaller one, filled with a dip, and placed it into the center of a serving platter, then filled half the platter with the cut vegetables from the second container.

Taking out cutlery from a drawer, he said to Karen, "I'm a night owl, so this is no bother for me."

"He likes to work at night and sleep in," Janice said. "The opposite of me."

"It's true," Fowler said with a shrug. "I do my best work long after the sun's gone down." He grinned at Janice. "At least our hours cross during part of the day, so we get the chance to argue about politics." He brought napkins, plates and cutlery to the table, then stood next to Janice's wheelchair, as though wondering what else he could do.

The microwave beeped. Fowler went behind the counter again and opened the oven door. Karen could smell the delicious aroma of what he'd prepared, and her immediate thought was, *Here I go again. Ready to stuff my face.* And then she thought, *What am I doing? What am I doing to myself? And to my marriage?* Searching for something to take her mind off these thoughts, she said to Fowler, "All those diplomas on the wall . . . just outside the kitchen . . . Are you some sort of doctor?"

"No," Fowler said "Those are Janice's. She has a PhD in genetics."

"What?" Karen turned to Janice, then immediately regretted her tone and look of surprise.

"There are ways a PhD can be earned without leaving the house," Janice said, shrugging. Then she added, "There's also a wall in our den filled with my father's plaques, for horticulture and writing . . . He's the real deep thinker in this family. I may have earned my doctorate, but that was only after he taught me *how* to earn it. How to think things through, make the right choices. How to believe I could do anything I put my mind to, if I could only find the courage."

Realizing that every assumption she'd made about Janice

had just been shattered, Karen found herself at a loss for words. But it was more than that, she knew. It was also Janice's remark about being able to do anything—if she could only find the courage. *Courage.* This was the second time tonight that word had struck her.

Fowler brought the platter over to the table. It now included meatballs, sesame chicken strips and red, green and yellow pepper strips, dotted with bite-size pieces of cauliflower. He placed the platter on the table and took his seat.

Leaning back in her chair, Karen glanced at Janice again, then once more lifted her eyes to the sign that read, *The Power of One Good Habit.*

—

# Five

Before reaching for any of the snacks, Karen sighed, knowing what she had to do. She cleared her throat. "Actually, I'd better call home first. May I use your phone?"

"Of course." Janice again pointed toward the door that led to the hallway. "It's just outside, on the small table."

Karen left the room. She tried to summon anger and failed, finding a mix of sadness and resignation instead. Gary picked up the phone on the first ring. "Where the hell are you?"

Karen attempted to explain, to keep her voice calm, but Gary cut her off angrily, saying, "You're pushing me too far, Karen."

"This is not the time to discuss it, Gary. I just called to make sure you're going to—" But before she could say, "Let me in," Gary slammed down the phone.

*Damn you!* Karen thought. *Why do you have to be so stubborn! All I did was stick up for my right to not be insulted.*

She returned to the kitchen and took her seat. For a few seconds there was an uncomfortable silence. Janice, looking concerned, said, "Is everything okay?"

Karen shook her head, her lips pressed into a line. "It's my husband Gary. He's hot-tempered, and once he gets fired up, it takes him a while to cool down."

"That can't be easy."

"It isn't." Karen reached for a chicken strip, adding, "We've been arguing for months now, ever since the baby was born. I wish there was something I could do—just snap my fingers and make everything better. But I can't. And I can't even put all the blame on Gary, because it's my fault too."

"What do you mean?" Janice asked.

Karen took a bite of the chicken strip and pointed at the platter of snacks. "This is the problem. Food. My weight. No matter what the argument is about, it always ends up being about that—the fact that I have no self-control."

To Karen's surprise, Fowler said, "That's not true."

"No. That isn't the way it works," Janice added.

But Karen, feeling a fresh rush of emotion, put the balance of the chicken strip onto her plate and said, "It's ruining our marriage. It's making him hate me. But I try!"

"I'm sure you do," Janice said.

Karen looked at Fowler for a moment and then turned back to Janice. "And then sometimes I think he's supposed to love me for who I am. The person inside this body. Why do *I* have to struggle to lose weight? Live on lettuce and carrots for the rest of my life? *He* wouldn't do it. I know him."

"Have you tried telling him that?" Janice asked. "The way you just told us?" She placed her small hands on the table.

"I'm not telling him anything!" Karen replied, her anger rising again. "He locked me out, can you believe it? Locked me and his son out of the house, just because I can't get my weight under control." She looked into Janice's eyes, then sighed. "I'm sorry. I'm sure you don't want to hear this."

"I'm a good listener," Janice said.

Karen reached out and touched her hand. Then she took a deep breath, and said, "You've both been so kind. And I really thank you for that . . . But I think it's time for me to leave."

"Where will you go?"

Karen had no answer.

Fowler said, "You're more than welcome to stay here for the night."

"Oh, no, I couldn't," Karen answered quickly.

Fowler didn't press her. Instead he said, "Then I can give you a lift somewhere, if that'll help."

"Maybe that will help," Karen said. Standing again, she added, "We've only been here a short time, just since Gary's transfer, and we don't know many people yet. But I have a friend at work—Sue. We've gotten quite close. I'm sure she'll let me spend the night at her place."

She gestured that she'd be back in a moment and again went to the telephone. But after getting Sue's voicemail, she put the phone down and walked back into the kitchen. She shook her head, saying, "She's not home," and remained standing. She was not looking forward to a night in the woods.

But Janice quickly cut into her thoughts. "Then it's settled. You'll stay here."

This time Karen hesitated. If she were alone, she knew, she might say yes instantly. But she was with Gabe, and though Janice and Fowler had reacted to her plight in the way only good neighbors would, they were still strangers.

Odd strangers.

Janice, picking up on Karen's reluctance, said, "I know you've just met us, and I suppose you could say we're a little different."

"No, really, it's not that."

Janice smiled. "Well, we *are* different. *I'm* different. And we're obviously not used to company. But if you could see past my appearance, past my father's eccentricities, we'd really love to have you be our guest. It would be no problem at all. The spare room's been ready for years." She laughed lightly.

Karen glanced at Fowler. He was staring at Janice, his eyes moist, his expression showing nothing but appreciation and pride. Karen said, "Well, okay then. Yes. Thank you. I would—we would—love to stay. And I can't tell you how grateful I am for the invitation."

Fowler smiled. "Excellent! Then it's settled. I'll just go get the blankets, then come back for Gabe." He stepped from the room.

Karen could see that Janice's eyes too had grown moist. She nodded at her and whispered, "Thank you."

Her own voice a whisper, Janice said, "No. I'm the one who should thank you."

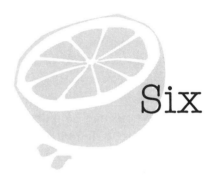

# Six

Karen awoke to sun shining through sheer curtains. It took a moment for her to orient herself, to re-member that this small neat room with the double bed and maple bureau was in Fowler's house. She looked over the side of the bed to see Gabe in his cradle, staring back at her, and whispered, "Good morning." Then, pushing her head deeper into the pillow, she sighed and replayed the events of the night before.

She was thankful it was Monday, so she didn't have to work—and Gary did. He would already be gone by the time she got home. For an instant she wondered if she would still be locked out, then dismissed that thought: Gary might be stubborn and insensitive about her weight, but he wasn't vengeful. And though she knew that last night's episode had brought their relationship to a new low, she thought—and hoped—that it could also be a starting-point from which to rebuild. She decided to look at it in that light, and try to get Gary to see it the same way.

Her thoughts shifted to who she was with, her unusual neighbors, and to a renewed appreciation for Janice.

Gabe let out a short, loud, insistent cry, and began waving his arms. Karen clumsily swung her legs off the side of the bed. Even that simple movement made her remember how graceful she'd been when she was sixty pounds lighter. She lifted Gabe into her arms and pressed her lips against his cheek, whispering, "I love you." Then she carried him over to the window and drew aside the curtain.

Fowler's garden was an immaculate sweep of color. Deep blues, intense reds. A painting of flowerbeds and winding pathways screened by a dense curtain of shrubbery and trees. Karen's eyes widened at both the vista and its seclusion. What she was seeing was only minutes from her own backyard, but completely hidden from its view. It's true, she thought, he *has* created a world of his own here.

She turned from the window and caught her reflection in a mirror on the bedroom door. Once again she felt the knot in her gut tighten.

All Karen could see was a pear-shaped figure with a heavy double chin. *You're right, Gary,* she thought. *It's me. You married someone thin, and no matter how much I try, I can't seem to change back.* But she forced these thoughts from her mind, knowing she had to get home as soon as possible to change and feed Gabe. She crossed the room, the baby still in her arms, and opened the door. Sitting on a chair in the hall was a stack of diapers. *I don't believe this,* she thought, her heart lifting at the kindness.

"Good morning," Janice said when Karen, a freshly changed Gabe in her arms, stepped into Fowler's restaurant a few minutes later.

This morning Janice wore a crisp white blouse. Instead of her blanket, she had on a long blue skirt that ended at her tiny feet. She touched the lever on her wheelchair and moved herself up to the table. A newspaper was spread out and another book, filled with mathematical symbols, was propped open against the fruit bowl. At the back of the room, Courage busily ate from a bowl set on a shelf a foot off the floor.

"Good morning," Karen said. "Thank you for the diapers . . ." Her eyes widened as she saw what else was waiting for her. "Oh, no! You shouldn't have . . . "

At the other end of the table were assorted jars of baby food and cereal, a bottle, colored spoons and a baby seat.

"I'll pay you back as soon—" Karen began.

Janice, smiling, shook her head. "Don't worry about the money."

"How could you even have thought of this?" Karen asked. "Gary would never have figured it out." She lifted Gabe into the baby seat and buckled him in, then reached for a jar of food and the spoons.

"It was my father's idea," Janice said, watching as Karen began to feed Gabe. "He's just not your typical kind of person. Somehow he always manages to be a little ahead of the curve."

"What do you mean?" Karen asked, noticing that Janice's appearance, even the sound of her voice, didn't feel quite as harsh to her as they had the night before.

"I mean, he has this ability to be a half-dozen steps ahead of everyone else, in whatever field interests him. Whether it's gardening or nutrition or philosophy." Janice reached out and touched the baby's foot, holding it for a moment, delight in her smile.

Karen smiled in response, then glanced at the book leaning against the fruit bowl and read the chapter title out loud: "Triangulating an n-Dimensional Cube."

"One of my hobbies," Janice said, "Trying to work out unsolved mathematical problems. I like the way they twist my mind, take me away from genetics. My father calls the work I do on the blackboard in the living room Chinese cooking."

Karen laughed. "It looks that way to me, too." Then, her

eyes falling once again on the sign on the wall, she asked, "What's the Power of One Good Habit?"

For a moment Janice didn't reply, then she said, slowly, "It's . . . a way of life. Something my father developed."

"A way of life?" Karen repeated, wiping a spill from Gabe's chin.

Janice nodded. "Actually, it's more something that fits into your life, without disrupting it." A moment later she added, "You know, you're the first person to ever ask what it means."

"What!" Karen laughed. "How could anyone see that sign and *not* ask what it means?"

Janice closed the newspaper and put it aside. "Because no one else has ever seen it. We don't have many visitors. In fact . . . we don't have any." Then she added, quickly, "The Power of One Good Habit—I must have begun hearing that phrase when I was eleven or twelve, maybe fifteen years ago."

"You're . . . twenty-seven?"

"Twenty-six."

Karen stared at Janice for a moment. Then she looked at the sign again, and at the trousers. "Were those your father's?"

Janice nodded.

"You mean, he was once that big?"

Again Janice nodded.

Karen shook her head. "I don't know how some people do it. Go on a diet and lose all that weight, and keep it off. I start a new diet every few months . . . "

"Diets aren't the answer," Janice said, touching Gabe's foot once again. "That's not how he lost his weight. Look in the cupboard behind you."

Karen offered Gabe a final spoonful of food, which he refused. Then she turned and opened the cupboard behind her chair. Inside were four shelves tightly packed with books. With just a glance at the titles, she could see they were all diet books.

"That's where my father keeps his diet book collection—

and he's read every one of them," Janice said. "Sometimes because he wanted to lose weight, and sometimes because he just wanted to see what new gimmick was currently making the rounds."

"I've read a lot of these books, too," Karen said. "And I'm still overweight."

"That's because diets don't work," Janice answered. "And the reason they don't work is that their approach is wrong. They try to tell you what to do, put you into the diet mentality of anxiety and guilt."

"Then what *does* work?"

"Just basic information, beginning with why you're overweight, and how to protect yourself from that. But I'd better let my father tell you about it. He has a knack for taking complexities and turning them into simple, commonsense truths—in a way most people can't."

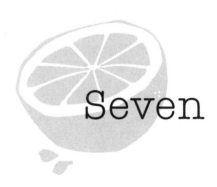

# Seven

"Good morning," Fowler said, just then stepping into the restaurant.

"Good morning," Karen answered. "And thank you for all this," she added, indicating the baby supplies on the table. "It's exactly what we needed." She gave Gabe the plastic spoon to play with, and he immediately brought it to his mouth.

"My pleasure," Fowler replied. Walking to the cooking area, he asked, "Tea or coffee?"

"Coffee," Janice answered.

"Coffee for me, too," Karen said. "But I should be going soon. I know Gary will be waiting to hear from me."

"You can always call him from here," Janice said.

"No. I don't think so. This isn't the place to talk about what happened last night . . . or to get another insult about my weight." She sighed and shook her head slowly, saying,

"Last night he called my weight his punishment for marrying me."

Janice said, quickly, "He can't mean that!"

"I don't know if he meant it, not exactly, but I do know what he means. I'm just not able to get my weight under control, no matter how hard I try. There are times when even I think there must be something wrong with me."

"There's nothing wrong with you!" Janice protested.

Karen shrugged and continued. "I know I'm a bright woman, and for three days a week I handle a responsible job—I manage the accounting department for a restaurant supply company. I'm valuable to them, I know that. And they prove it to me by paying me well and letting me work under the conditions I need so I can also spend time with Gabe. I know all that, tell it to myself. Then I hear Gary, or just step in front of a mirror, and I know there must be something wrong."

Fowler brought three coffees to the table and went back behind the counter. The two women murmured their thanks.

"I *will* lose the weight, though, I know it," Karen said, taking a sip of the coffee. But even as Janice began to nod in agreement, she shook her head. "No, I won't. Who am I kidding? I've tried enough times to know it'll never come off. For me, losing weight is only a dream. I'm someone who doesn't even have to eat to gain extra pounds. Just the smell of burgers and fries does it. And I can't go on another diet! I can't even face that thought." Gabe's eyes were beginning to close. Karen took the spoon from his hand, then held his hand for a moment, stroking the back of it with her thumb.

Fowler returned to the table with three glasses of water, each with a slice of lemon in it.

Karen said, looking at him, "Janice said you were once overweight, too."

Fowler sat and leaned back in his chair. "No, that's not quite true. I'm still overweight. What you're looking at is an overweight person in a thin body. And I'm proud to be that way. Not ashamed to say I have a weight problem. And, like you, I also gain weight with just the smell of burgers and fries. But I have the problem under control."

"Because of that?" Karen asked, pointing at the sign. "The Power of One Good Habit?"

Fowler nodded.

"The Power of One Good Habit isn't a diet," Janice said, "but it did solve his weight problem."

"I used the concept behind it to think it all through," Fowler said, taking a sip of his coffee. "To think through why I was overweight. Think it through carefully and common-sense-fully. It let me define the problem, so I could then learn the information I needed to solve it."

Karen said, "I'd love to not have to diet again. When I was thirty pounds overweight, I starved myself down fifteen pounds—then gained back twenty! Then I lost the twenty on a low-carb diet because that's all everyone was talking about—"

"That won't work," Janice said. "Not in the long run."

"You're right," Karen agreed. "When I couldn't stand not being able to eat half the foods I loved, I gained the twenty back—and more!" She took one last swallow of her coffee and stood, saying, "I'm sorry, but I really have to go." She began to unbuckle Gabe from the baby seat.

"Will you come back?" Janice asked.

"Yes. I'd like that."

"You can bring Gabe," Janice said. "We can talk again."

Fowler, also standing, said, "How about tomorrow? Can you come for lunch?"

After only a second's hesitation, Karen said, "Lunch sounds perfect. Thank you for the invitation—and for everything."

—

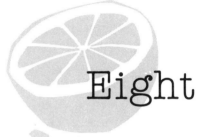

# Eight

This time, Karen took the side street that joined her development to the old two-lane highway running past Fowler's front door. The day was warm and the sky clear, but her thoughts about Gary were anything but sunny.

He telephoned from his office only minutes after she got into the townhouse. At first he was repentant, apologizing for losing his temper and locking her out, saying he didn't know why he had done it and promising it would never happen again. But after asking about the neighbors she'd stayed with, and hearing about Fowler's eccentricities and Janice's condition, and then about the sign on the wall, he'd blown up again, saying, "How could you have stayed there? Especially with Gabe!"

He hadn't let her get in even a single word after that, shouting, "If you want to walk the streets, do it! If you want to go to some fleabag hotel, you can do that too! But you keep my son away from people like that!" Then he'd hung up.

He came home late, without explanation, and spent the evening in bad-tempered silence.

It was only as she came up Fowler's front walk the next day, though, that Karen realized what was bothering her most. It wasn't Gary's words—as much as his tone. A tone, she felt, that was so foul and angry, that it should not be part of any marriage.

Fowler opened the door. The expression on his face when he saw Karen was one of complete pleasure. "Hello! Hello! Hello!" he said, exuberantly shaking her hand in both of his, getting a laugh from Karen. Then he turned his welcome to Gabe in the stroller. He called out Gabe's name, feigning complete surprise, then made a face designed to make a child laugh. Gabe bounced in his seat and held his hands out to Fowler. Fowler lifted him from the stroller.

Janice, staying well in the house so she could not be seen from the front door, smiled broadly and said excitedly, "Welcome again, Karen!"

They went to the kitchen, and Karen was surprised how wonderfully at home she suddenly felt. But as Fowler strapped Gabe into the child seat he'd bought for him the night before, Karen took her cell phone from her bag and said, "If I get a call, please don't listen to what I'm going to say, because I'm not supposed to be here."

Janice, reaching for Gabe's hand, said, "If your husband calls, you say whatever you have to. Don't worry about us."

Fowler agreed, then asked, "What would you like for lunch? Any requests?"

"Oh, I'm going to leave that up to you," Karen said. "You're the expert."

"Sounds good to me," Fowler replied, stepping into the cooking area. On the counter was a tray of assorted cut vegetables spread invitingly around a dip. Fowler reached for a piece of green pepper.

Karen, walking up to the counter, asked, "Can I help with

anything?" She smiled. "I worked my way through college as a waitress, so if you need me to balance a couple of meals in one hand and a pot of coffee in the other, I'm a pro. I even worked in the kitchen. In fact, that was the best part of the job."

"An assistant with experience?" Fowler said. "I'd never refuse an offer like that."

At the table, Janice was stroking Gabe's arm and talking softly to him. Gabe wore a wide, toothless smile. A math book and assorted papers lay on the table, but for the moment Janice was ignoring them.

Fowler grinned at Karen and said, "Looks like Gabe's found a new friend." Then he filled three glasses with water and dropped a slice of lemon into each. Stepping around the counter, he brought one of the glasses to Janice, saying to Karen, "How about something quick and easy, one of our favorites? I call it Kickin' Chicken with Fries, sort of."

"Sort of?"

"You'll see what I mean," Fowler said, stepping back behind the counter.

"Anything with potatoes sounds good to me," Karen said. "I love potatoes. I love fries. Just tell me what to do."

"Okay. Why don't you start by peeling the spuds? Say about twelve."

From the table Janice said, "Twelve potatoes for three people? I guess we're in for some of my father's kind of cooking."

Karen smiled quizzically. She took a good swallow of the water with lemon, set the glass on the counter, and got down to work. But, glancing at the sign on the wall again, she couldn't resist saying, "You talked about the Power of One Good Habit, and said it wasn't a diet. But I still don't know what it is, what that sign means."

Fowler had turned the oven on to preheat, then took two packages of chicken breasts out of the refrigerator. Now he was trimming all the skin and visible fat from the chicken. "That sign," he said, "is the way I remind myself how powerful one habit can be. How, when we adopt one seemingly insignificant change into our everyday lives, the result, over time, can surpass all expectations. And when we add one habit onto another, and then another, the result can be nothing less than life-changing." He worked the knife for a moment before saying, "That's what I did. By adopting eight core habits, one after the other, I changed my life from one that promoted weight gain to one that now promotes health and weight loss. That sign reminds me how powerful each one of those eight habits is, and how they're all, now, an integral part of my life."

"Tell her your tire analogy," Janice said, looking up from playing with Gabe. Her finger was once again in the baby's grasp.

Fowler grinned. "That's the way I first explained the Power of One Good Habit to Janice, by comparing it to a tire, like one of the tires on my old car. But instead of an engine making this tire roll, its power comes from a tiny pulse of courage."

*Courage again,* Karen thought.

"And that tiny pulse of courage," Fowler continued, "that small amount we need just to begin the first small change, gets the tire rolling, gets the habit forming, and moves us forward a step or two along our chosen journey. Then another pulse of courage, with another small change, zaps that tire again, taking us even further ahead. And it's those small forward steps, steps that on their own seem insignificant, that keep the tire rolling indefinitely. They not only get us to our goal—they keep us there."

"And the power of those eight habits is available to all of us," Janice added, not taking her eyes off Gabe as she spoke.

"It is," Fowler agreed. "But that doesn't mean we'll all apply the habits." He picked a piece of red pepper from the bowl of cut vegetables on the counter, dipped it into the dip, popped it into his mouth, then washed it down with a good swallow of his water with lemon. Seeing that Karen had finished peeling the potatoes, he took a large mixing bowl off the shelf and said, "Now give the spuds a quick rinse, then cut them into wedges and put them into this bowl, and I'll show you how I prepare them."

While Karen was doing that, Fowler began combining the ingredients he would need to coat the chicken breasts, beginning with salsa and Dijon mustard.

"I don't understand," Karen said. "If the power of those eight habits is available to all of us, then why is it that only some of us will be able to apply them?"

"Because," Fowler answered, "most of us have been brainwashed by the diet industry into believing that the only way to lose weight is by buying into whatever newfangled diet they're currently selling. The latest fad that turns our lives upside down. The fad we'll all jump on—then all fail at." He laughed. "The last thing the diet industry wants is for us to realize just how powerful a few simple practical habits can be, because there's no profit for them in that. They don't want us to know that even a single simple habit—a habit that on its own seems insignificant—once integrated into your life, will have a life-changing impact."

Karen finished rinsing the potatoes then began cutting them into wedges. She nodded, thinking about what Fowler was saying.

Fowler, mixing his ingredients in a bowl, said, "But the diet industry doesn't control all of us. So some people, like me, through trial and error, will discover this knowledge on their own. And then others will simply learn it from those of us who've figured it out. But most people are so busy just getting from one day to the next, just living their lives, that they don't have the time or energy to do either."

Karen, brow furrowed, put the last of the cut potatoes into the bowl. Fowler handed her a baking sheet and said, "Now drizzle some olive oil over them, toss them to spread the oil, then season them with a dash of salt and lots of pepper, garlic powder and oregano. Then put them on this baking sheet and we'll pop them in the oven."

"Just a dash of salt?" Karen said.

"Just a dash. Because no salt would leave it tasteless."

"Because of my egging him on," Janice said, turning to Karen, "my father discovered that when it comes to salt, a little goes a long way, especially when combined with all his other spices."

Fowler laughed, saying, "Don't spill all our secrets!"

Karen began following Fowler's directions, but her mind was still on his explanation of the Power of One Good Habit. "Okay," she said finally, turning to Fowler. "In your tire analogy you talked about a tiny pulse of courage moving us forward on our journey . . . But . . . I don't know what you mean by *journey*."

Fowler had placed the chicken breasts in a baking dish and was now pouring the salsa mixture over them. "When I talk about journeys, I mean our journeys in life. And for me, taking a life journey, like stopping smoking or drinking or—"

"Eating?" Karen asked.

"No. We all have to eat," Fowler said, putting the chicken in the oven and closing the door. "What I mean is eating healthy, eating in a way that will allow you to get your weight under control and keep it there. And that's the journey I think of most when I talk about the Power of One Good Habit."

"He calls that journey a war," Janice said.

"That's right," Fowler agreed. "A war—one that can only be won through knowledge." He snapped his fingers, made a beeline for the freezer and took out a package of asparagus spears. He placed the spears in a shallow pan of water and set it on the stove.

"A war won through knowledge," Karen repeated.

"That's it," Fowler said. He swallowed down the last of his water with lemon and watched as Karen spiced the potatoes, then, while helping her spread them evenly on the baking sheet, said, "The trouble most people have with fighting the war to lose weight, to regain their health, is that they don't *know* they're in a war. And if they do realize there's a war going on around them, then they don't know who the enemy is. And if they get a feel for the enemy, then they don't have the information they need to defeat it."

Karen said slowly, "The Power of One Good Habit begins with a tiny pulse of courage, which, combined with the right information, lets you defeat the enemy."

"Exactly," Fowler said as he placed the potatoes in the oven.

Karen's expression grew suddenly somber. "Well, in my case, with my war against being overweight, I know who the enemy is. Me."

"You're not your own enemy," Janice said.

"Janice is right," Fowler said. "When it comes to being overweight, no one is their own enemy. Not unless they want to be." He set the timer on the oven and said, "The cutlery and napkins are in the top drawer, so if you can set the table, I'll get the salad going. And we'll also need refills of our water with lemon."

While Karen set the table, Fowler took a bag of store-bought prewashed greens from the refrigerator, poured a good serving into three oversized salad bowls, then topped them with grape tomatoes, sliced cucumber and a lowfat dressing. He put the bowls back into the refrigerator, checked how the asparagus was coming, saw he was able to easily pierce the vegetables with a fork, and drained them. Then he placed them in a covered glass dish and put them on top of the stove to stay warm.

Turning to Karen he said, "Okay, we've got at least a half hour until the chicken and potatoes are ready, and I've got an orchid that's been crying out for weeks to be repotted. A real beaut, a Vanda, with hanging roots that are over four feet long. So an extra pair of hands would be very helpful. What do you say? Ever repot an orchid?"

"No. Never. And I'd love to help!" Karen said excitedly. "Your plants are just amazing, and I want to know your secret. You'll just have to tell me exactly what to do."

"I'll watch Gabe," Janice said, "while the two of us watch you."

*  *  *

"It's because you're an expert," Karen said to Fowler as they stepped back into the kitchen after repotting the orchid. She was holding Gabe in his baby chair, and she placed him on the table, saying, "Boy, something smells great!"

"It's the chicken," Janice said, steering her wheelchair into the room. Courage, as usual, was right beside her.

"I'm not an expert," Fowler said. "Just an enthusiastic amateur who isn't afraid to figure out the hows and whys of whatever interests me." He put a couple of dog biscuits into Courage's bowl, then went back behind the counter and opened the oven door. "Looking good," he said, reaching for the oven mitts. He took out both the chicken and the potatoes, placing them on top of the stove, then took down three plates from the cupboard.

"What should I do?" Karen asked, stepping into the cooking area.

"Just get the salad bowls from the fridge. I can handle the rest."

While Karen got the salad bowls, Fowler put a generous serving of the asparagus on each plate, then added one chicken breast and a handful of potato wedges. Most of the chicken and potatoes he'd cooked was left in their baking dishes. He brought the plates to the table.

Karen kissed the top of Gabe's head and placed him in his baby seat to one side of the table, next to where she was sitting.

Fowler sat, saying to Karen, "Eat! Dig in! Enjoy! You're not going to find any formality in my restaurant."

"I will! And thank you so much for inviting us over." She cut off a piece of the chicken and tasted it, then said, "This is excellent!"

"It's one of our standards," Janice said. "Something we always enjoy."

Fowler said, "I like it because it's quick and always tasty and takes absolutely no thought."

44

Karen nodded, but her mind was on the potatoes she had prepared under Fowler's supervision. She held one up with her fork, "These are really good, too."

"Thank you," Fowler said. "They're one of my favorites. My unfried French fries."

"They do taste like fries, don't they?" Karen said. "Only better—tangier."

"He makes them by the bagful," Janice said, "We both love them. For breakfast, lunch and dinner."

"Snacks too," Fowler added. "I can eat them cold—or warm them in the microwave or oven. Potatoes are a gift of the gods, and meant to be eaten—"

He was interrupted by a loud squeal from Gabe. The baby was looking at Janice, smiling broadly, arms waving excitedly.

Janice laughed with obvious delight.

Fowler laughed along with her.

Courage stood and barked.

The cell phone rang.

—

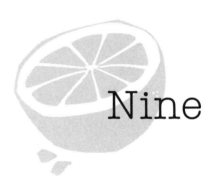

# Nine

It was three days before Karen saw Fowler and Janice again. Once more she stood on their back porch with Gabe in her arms. The porch light was off, the back of the house dark.

She hated being here like this, but hadn't known what else to do. She had to get away, and this was the only place she felt comfortable going.

Gary's attitude had grown worse as the days had gone by. Karen had tried to understand him; she told herself that his anger was temporary, that it was the pressures of his new job, a new sales territory, the new house, the baby.

But he refused to discuss it. Told her he was tired of talking.

When he'd called her cell phone during lunch, the first words he'd said were, "Where are you? And don't lie to me!"

"Gary . . ."

"You're back there with those freaks, aren't you?"

"Yes," she said softly. Then she immediately added, "No! I mean, Gary, you have it all wrong! There's absolutely nothing—" But the connection had already gone dead.

She left the house quickly then, knowing that for her marriage's sake she could not see Fowler and Janice again.

But what began with that phone call, turned into something that had never happened before, something Karen would never have dreamed could happen: three days of silence, interrupted only by insults.

She did what she had to do—her job, the housekeeping, looking after Gabe. She waited for Gary to come around, for him to see his own lack of reason, to show some compassion. Karen tried to talk to him, but it didn't work. Nothing worked.

Then tonight, while Gary was in the recliner watching baseball on TV and she sat on the sofa reading, he'd finally spoken. "What's wrong with you?" He muted the volume on the television. "Can't you figure out what the problem is?"

"I know what the problem is," Karen said calmly, looking at Gary's thick, round face.

"Oh? You do? And what is it?"

"The problem is me."

"Well, you're right there!"

"The problem is I can't take care of myself. Of my weight. I know that." Then she said, "And I can't find any courage."

"Courage? What do you mean? Courage to do what?"

"I don't know. Something. Everything." It was this word that had stuck with her. Out of all that Janice and Fowler had said, this was the word that continually ran through her mind. *Courage.* A tiny amount of courage, just enough to take you to the next step. She could feel Gary's anger build, see his arms and fists tensing. She thought, *I may not be the same woman you married, Gary, but you're not the same man either. That man began to pack his things after Gabe was conceived. And had left by the time he was born.*

She took a deep breath. "If there's something wrong with

me, Gary, then what about you? You chose me. And had a baby with me."

* * *

Though the porch light was off, Karen could see there were lights on in the house. Courage pressed his nose against the screen. Karen whispered, "Courage." Then Fowler stepped into the doorway, clearly surprised to see her.

"I'm sorry," she whispered. "I didn't know where else—"

"Don't be. It's all right."

He led her into the house and lifted Gabe into the baby seat that had become a fixture on the large kitchen table. Karen heard Janice call from down the hall and Fowler went to her.

He returned in just a few moments, followed by Janice in her wheelchair. She was wearing pajamas, her expression a mixture of happiness and unease.

Fowler put the kettle on for tea.

Stopping her wheelchair next to Karen, Janice said, "Do you want to talk about it?"

Karen shook her head. She was fighting back frustration and anger, and wasn't sure which emotion fit where. She said to Janice, "No. I just appreciate you being here."

"That's what friends are for," Janice answered.

* * *

Karen woke the next morning before either Janice or Fowler. When she stepped into the kitchen with Gabe in her arms she found another assortment of baby supplies waiting on the table. She stared at them a moment, then began to look for a piece of paper and a pen or pencil.

Janice steered her chair into the room.

Karen turned to her. "I was going to just sneak out," she said. "Leave a thank-you note."

"Sneak out? Why?" Gabe stretched his hands toward Janice, and she exclaimed, "He recognizes me!"

Karen nodded. She was dreading her next words.

Janice clearly sensed that something was wrong. "Why were you going to sneak out? Is it because you're afraid of Gary?"

"No, of course not."

"Then what is it?"

Karen sighed. "I'm not afraid of Gary. I'm afraid of *losing* him. And he's upset with me because I was here. Because I came back here . . . and now I'm back again."

Janice looked directly at Karen and said, her voice firm, "Please, have a seat for a minute. There's something I want to say."

Karen, with Gabe in her arms, sat at the table.

"You've said your marriage is in trouble because of your weight," Janice said.

Karen nodded. "It is. Gary hates it. And I hate it too."

"All right, then. My father's found a way to solve that problem."

Karen winced and shook her head, feeling herself fall with a thud into a new bout of hopelessness at just the thought of another diet. Another failure. After a moment's silence, she said, "I can't. I'm not ready. I'm not prepared." She knew she had to psych herself up first. Be in a state of mind to push her willpower to the limit. To not eat carbohydrates or fat or any of the foods she craved for as long as possible—until she slipped—then fell.

"But you need it now," Janice said.

Just then, Fowler walked into the room. "Good morning!"

Janice turned to him. "Karen says she's not ready for the Power of One Good Habit. That she's not sure about it."

For a moment Fowler remained quiet. Then he said to Karen, "Well, to be honest, I'd rather hear you say you're not sure about it than hear you say you're gung-ho and can't

49

wait to have your life changed. That shows me you've got a healthy amount of skepticism."

Janice looked as though she wanted to say something, but didn't.

"On the other hand," Fowler continued, "the only thing we've told you was that to win the war against being over-weight, all you're missing is knowledge. Knowledge we have. And that's all there is. No magic pill. Nothing to buy." He shrugged. "So maybe your hesitation has less to do with good, healthy skepticism and more to do with something else."

Karen's jaws tightened. She took a deep breath, felt her anger rise. *Why are you pressuring me, Fowler? If I want to go on a diet, I'll do it myself. My way!* Then she thought, *They just don't understand.*

She sighed. "Fowler, unlike you, I'm the type of person who fails at diets. Always. That's why I'm so big. So if you try to teach me what you know, I won't understand what you're saying, or I won't be able to do whatever it is you expect of me. I won't be able to stick with it. And I'll fail again. And this time I'll not only disappoint myself and Gary, but also you."

Janice, with her brow still creased in thought, said, "Are you saying, then, that you're afraid to simply listen and learn about the eight habits, because you're afraid you'll fail at them?"

"Janice, we have to respect Karen's decision," Fowler said gently.

"*You* might have to," Janice answered, "but *I* don't." Her husky voice suddenly rose as she said to Karen, "Do you know I was supposed to be dead twenty-six years ago? And then, after twenty-five or thirty operations before I turned five, my father was still told my chances of seeing ten were nonexistent? And even now, the best the doctors can do is say they don't know why I'm still here, that my father should be prepared for me to not wake up tomorrow morning or the one after that!"

50

She fixed her gaze on Karen. "And can you imagine how it feels to look the way I do, to have to hide in this house? Flinch from the doorway even from the postman? Know I'll never have a husband, a child, the way you do? Never have even a chance at that kind of life, that kind of love?"

She paused, and Karen was trying to think of something to say when Janice resumed. "My father says I should respect your decision to not try to take control of your situation, to not show the strength your son, your perfect baby boy, should be able to rely on. Well, I don't respect it. In fact, it makes me livid to think that *just the thought of failure* is enough to stop anyone from having the courage to take a step forward."

Her small hands were balled into fists. She took a deep breath, then shouted, "You said you wanted to sneak out. Well, okay! Go!" And with that she backed her chair from the table and maneuvered herself out of the room.

—

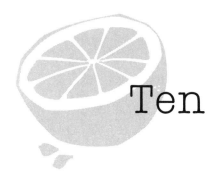

# Ten

They both sat motionless. Fowler looked stunned. "She never told me that before."

Karen was breathing heavily, as though she'd been running. She lowered her head, felt shame and suddenly realized what hopelessness really meant. She lifted her eyes to Fowler. He was still staring at the door. She whispered to him, "Please watch Gabe," and, handing the baby to him, went to find Janice.

Janice was in the den she shared with Fowler, facing the curtained window flanked by their two large desks, each a jumble of papers and books, a computer and accessories and snakes of cables.

To her right was a wall filled with Fowler's gardening plaques and ribbons. The other walls held bookshelves crammed with texts and magazines and bound manuscripts. This room too was filled with plants.

"Janice," Karen whispered.

Janice said nothing. Made no movement.

"Janice, I'm sorry."

Janice slowly turned her chair around.

"I never meant to hurt you," Karen said. "I was only being honest, and weak, and I'm sorry."

In an angry but even voice, Janice said, "Sorry? For whom? For me? Or for yourself? Because if it's for me, don't be. I long ago accepted that I can't change my appearance, so I ignore it and work on what I can change—my health, my mind. Because, as human beings, that's what we do. That's our function. Beyond the genetic level of reproduction, our function in this life is to progress—physically, intellectually, and spiritually. No matter what, we can't stand still."

"I know you're right," Karen said, her eyes filling with tears.

"I used to look at the eight habits as complete in themselves," Janice continued. "But I was wrong. I see that now. There's a step outside them that has to be taken first. A step we have to provide for ourselves, from within."

Karen wiped her eyes. "It's . . . fear," she said. "Repeated failure. That's what's holding me back." The one word that kept swirling through her mind was *courage*. She lowered her head, took a deep breath, then whispered in a small voice, "Help me, Janice. Please?"

They returned to the kitchen together. Gabe was buckled into his baby seat, Fowler seated in front of him. Janice said, "Karen asked me to help her take the first step toward making the Power of One Good Habit a part of her life. I told her I would help, as much as I could. I gave her a notebook so she could start a journal."

Fowler nodded, but Karen could see his concern was still for Janice. He questioned her with his eyes until he was satisfied with what he saw, and only then did he allow himself to relax and say, "Asking for help *is* the first step."

Karen looked at him. "You mean I've taken the first step?"

"Of course. Asking for help is the necessary first step to

making the eight habits work. The first step to finding the information." Again he looked at Janice, then he stood and walked behind the counter and began filling the coffeemaker.

Janice steered her wheelchair to the table.

Fowler prepared three coffees and three glasses of water with lemon and brought them over on a tray. He took his seat. For a moment the only one who spoke was Gabe, babbling happily to himself.

Karen, looking at Fowler, said, "I'll try to make this work. Try as hard as I've ever tried anything."

She was being honest, she knew. But not forthright. And that was the best she could do. She'd try. She just had no faith she would succeed. She held up the spiral-bound notebook Janice had given her. "Janice said I should make notes—about each of the eight habits. I'm going to write it all down, try to understand everything."

Fowler said, "The eight core habits are as simple as your ABCs. Once you begin, each one will pull you along. Just let it happen. Take in the information, go where the information points, listen to your head and you can't fail."

Karen began to say, "I've dieted—"

"Let me say it again," Fowler interrupted. "The Power of One Good Habit is *not* a diet—and it doesn't require a diet mentality. It's just basic knowledge that will show you how to look at your weight in a different way, from a different angle. It'll show you why you've lost control over your weight and don't even know it. Why all you know is that you're getting heavier. Why the whole country's getting heavier.

"After I've explained them to you, you'll see for yourself that you can't do the eight habits wrong, because with each habit everything is *right*. And you can't go *off* the habits once you begin using them, because they're not something you're *on*. And you'll never have to start the habits over, because they can't end. Once you start them, they can't end. Ever."

"It really *isn't* a diet, is it?" Karen said.

"No, the Power of One Good Habit isn't a diet. In fact, its primary goal isn't even to lose weight, although you *will* lose all the weight you need to. What the eight habits really do is return control of your health where it belongs—in your hands."

Karen, nodding her head, thought, *You make it sound so easy. Just listen to your words—and lose weight. But that's impossible, isn't it?* She laughed lightly, then said, "Okay, how do we start?"

"We start," Fowler said, "the way we start every morning. With breakfast."

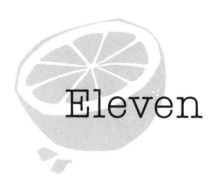

# Eleven

Karen said to Fowler, "This time I'm not even *asking* if I can help prepare breakfast."

"And this time," Janice said, "I'll officially baby-sit." She reached for a plastic turnip Fowler had bought for Gabe and held the toy out to the baby.

Karen stepped behind the counter with Fowler, thinking, *I'll do my best to learn the eight habits—and fail later. And knowing that in advance will take all the pressure and struggle out of it.* She thought briefly of the call she'd get from Gary when she got home, but for the moment pushed that inevitable confrontation from her mind.

"In the restaurant world," Fowler began, "there's a certain protocol that has to be followed. And it goes like this: I'm the chef, so I'm the boss. And starting now, you're the *sous-chef*, and that's French for 'when you work here, you're the gofer.'"

Karen laughed. "That's fine with me."

"Good. Now there's something else I have to tell you, and it's about the Power of One Good Habit."

"Okay."

"You see, I may know my stuff—I should, I've been learning and living it for the better part of two decades—but that doesn't mean I know how to teach it, so what I'm going to do is a lot of lip-flapping. About everything. And we'll see where that gets us."

Karen smiled and nodded.

"Now to our first order of business," Fowler said, looking over at Janice. "My staff and I need to know what you want for breakfast."

"Something fast and simple," Janice said, "because Karen has to go home and talk to her husband—then arrange to come back later for lunch."

Karen smiled and said, "You can count on that."

"So what do you want?" Fowler asked again.

"French toast."

"I love French toast," Karen said. "So does Gary. That's the problem for both of us: bread."

Fowler said, "There's no such thing as a problem food, be it bread or anything else." But before Karen could question this, he rapidly said, "Okay! Right now, we need eggs, milk and bread. Let's go, let's go, there're a hundred hungry people out there!" He grinned and, while Karen took the eggs and milk from the refrigerator, said, "The primary focus of the Power of One Good Habit is your health, and that's where it first takes effect. And if you have to lose weight for your health's sake—"

"I do."

"Then you will. But if you don't, the health effects will kick in anyway. The Power of One Good Habit will lower your cholesterol, lower your blood pressure, control your blood sugar and make you less susceptible to diabetes and heart disease and arthritis, and even some cancers."

"All that?" Karen asked, turning to him from the counter where she had placed the items from the refrigerator.

"All that, and more. And when it comes to weight, there's something else I want you to keep in mind. We're not concerned with pounds. What we really want is to lower our percentage of body fat, the amount of fat our bodies have compared to all the muscle and bones and everything else. That's the real weight goal. Because even someone who thinks their weight is fine, who looks like a million bucks in their clothes, can still have too much fat in their body, while a football player, some massive bruiser who clocks in at three hundred pounds, may be, fat-wise, perfect."

"So I have to work with percentages?"

"No."

"But you said—"

"There's no working with numbers at all. Not with any of the habits. In fact, you don't even have to weigh yourself."

Karen laughed. "I can't go without weighing myself! Especially if I'm losing weight."

"I know you can't. I can't either. But we really don't have to—because nothing about the eight habits works with specifics. And weighing yourself too often also leaves you open to getting depressed over a weight gain that isn't even true, because our weight can move up or down a pound or two or three from one day to the next, and have nothing to do with either gaining or losing fat."

"I didn't know that," Karen said.

"It's only the bigger picture that counts. Once a week. Every two weeks. Once a month."

From the table Janice said, "When my father was losing his weight, his goal was to be down one pound a week, and to keep track he used to weigh himself every Sunday morning. And nine out of ten Sundays he would be down that pound, until he had nothing left to lose."

Karen's eyes opened wide. But Fowler shrugged aside what Janice said by simply stating, "Every step in the right direction is a success in itself, and any progress is exceptional progress. And remember this, too: the best scale isn't a scale at all, it's your clothes. The scale may lie, but your clothes never do. Those old jeans, by the time I finally hung them on the wall, told me everything I needed to know. And the ones I'm wearing now do the same. They keep me on my toes." He grinned and, stepping to the counter, said, "Okay, I'll prepare the French toast while you make a fresh pot of coffee and set the table. Filters are over there, and the coffee's next to the coffeemaker." And, glancing back at the table, he added, "We'll also need three more glasses of water with lemon."

Karen refilled the coffeemaker, then brought the cutlery and napkins to the table. Meanwhile Fowler took a package of whole grain bread from the breadbox and placed it next to the eggs. He began cracking the eggs into a mixing bowl. Karen said, "French toast made with wheat bread? I never had that before."

"Not wheat bread," Fowler said. "Wheat bread is just white bread with added coloring."

"Excuse me?" Karen said

Janice laughed. "That's right. White bread is still made from wheat, so if it's colored brown, it's sometimes called wheat bread. The word you need to look for is *whole* wheat, or *whole* grain. That's the real deal." Then she added for Gabe, "Isn't that right?"

"And today," Fowler said, "you're in for an extra treat, because this bread isn't *just* whole wheat, it's whole multi-grain. That's whole wheat plus more."

"There's three different grains in that bread," Janice said, "including ground flax seed."

"Exactly," Fowler said. "And texture-wise, there's a huge difference from whole wheat. Whole wheat is nutritious, all right, but whole multi-grain is not only nutritious, it's especially tasty."

Janice said, "I got him to try whole multi-grain. In fact, it's me who gets him to try almost everything new."

"That's true," Fowler admitted. "If it wasn't for Janice's curious streak I'd never experience anything different. For years I was a white-bread-only kind of guy, just never adapted to whole wheat, even though Janice loved it. But once Janice got me to try whole multi-grain, I was sold." He lifted up a piece of the whole multi-grain bread. "Even if I tried, I couldn't do it better. And the taste is fantastic."

"It took a while," Janice said, "but I finally got him to see that variety in eating is truly the spice of life."

Fowler smiled.

"Quite the endorsement," Karen said. "After that I'm looking forward to tasting it." For a moment she watched as Fowler continued to crack the eggs into the mixing bowl, then she said to him, "What are you doing?"

"I'm preparing the eggs for the French toast."

"But the yolks . . . ?"

One by one, Fowler was dropping the egg whites into the mixing bowl and throwing the egg yolks into the garbage, until he came to the last two eggs. Only with those did he also include the yolk. He said, "This restaurant hasn't used the same number of egg yolks as egg whites in ten years—and it never will again."

"Sometimes he saves them for other things," Janice said. "Like the insect repellent he makes for his flowers."

"Waste not, want not," Fowler said.

Karen wrinkled her nose. "But won't the French toast look gross with only two yolks?" she asked.

"We'll just have to see about that," Fowler said. Then he quickly added, "In this restaurant, breakfast and fruit go to-gether, so pick out whatever you like from the fruit bowl, be generous, and let's make this meal kick!"

While Karen prepared the fruit, Fowler poured a splash of one-percent milk in with the eggs, beat the mixture well and began to soak the bread in it. Then he got a large frying pan from the cupboard and, after spraying it with oil from a pump sprayer, started to fry the bread.

When she was finished with the fruit, Karen brought the coffeepot and cups to the table, refilled the glasses with cold water and fresh slices of lemon, then lined up their three plates, each now adorned with orange wedges, strawberries and a slice of cantaloupe.

Fowler said, "We like our French toast with my special blueberry topping. In fact, we use that instead of syrup."

"Blueberry topping?" Karen said. "Sounds interesting. I'll have that, too."

"Great," Fowler said. He popped two cups of frozen berries into the microwave and left them until they first thawed, then cooked down to one cup of blueberry topping. Then, when the toast was ready, he put two slices onto each plate, alongside a couple of strips of lowfat cheddar cheese, shouted, "Pickup!" and he and Karen carried the plates and the topping to the table.

Gabe had tired of his turnip and was now testing the re-siliency of Janice's cheek. Janice said, "He doesn't know what he's touching—so it doesn't bother him."

"It shouldn't bother anyone," Karen said, before taking a bite of her French toast.

Janice was smiling. "How is it?"

"Excellent! The topping *and* the multi-grain bread."

"I like the light sweetness of the blueberries better than the heavy sweetness of syrup," Janice said.

"They're also filled with beneficial antioxidants," Fowler added. "Brain food, right?" he said, looking at Janice.

"Something like that," Janice said, smiling. Then, turning to Karen, she added, "Did you remember that my father used only two egg yolks to make the French toast?"

Karen's brows rose. "No. I forgot about that. They're—I mean, the color and taste are perfect!"

Fowler said, "Using fewer egg yolks *is* a part of the Power of One Good Habit, and the Power of One Good Habit *will* solve your weight problem, I'm sure of that. But a logical way to introduce you to it, before going into details like bread or egg yolks, is to first tell you why you're overweight."

Karen, digging heartily into her food, laughed. "Why I'm overweight? *This* is why I'm overweight! Because of my appetite."

"Really?" Fowler said. "Tell me, what would you do if Gabe didn't want to eat?"

"Well, I'd worry, of course."

"Right. And if it persisted?"

Karen shrugged. "I'd take him to the doctor."

"Exactly. And that's because having no appetite is a sign of poor health, while having a strong appetite is a sign of *good* health. You're not overweight because of your appetite. No one is."

"Then what is it?"

"Go ahead," Fowler said to Janice. "This is your field."

"The reason most people are overweight," Janice said, putting down her fork, "is because our bodies were designed for the way life was thousands of years ago, not for the way it is today. We were designed for a time when people had to *search* for their food. They had to gather it or hunt it or raise it themselves. Back then, people were on their own, in complete control of everything to do with eating. And they ate to sustain themselves. They ate to keep themselves healthy."

"You mean our food is too easy to get?" Karen asked.

"No," Janice said. "That's not it. The problem is that these days we've given the control of our food over to our modern culture. And for the most part, when it comes to food, our modern culture focuses on convenience, taste and appearance, and *not* on what's good for our health. And that's why there's a problem."

Fowler said, "It helps if you realize that there are three very different groups involved in producing the food we eat. First, there are the people who raise it for us, the farmers and ranchers and fishermen who give us all our fresh foods, all the meats and poultry and fish and vegetables and fruits and grains. And they're the wonders of the world! Bless them all.

"Then there's the second group, and this group consists of some excellent health-minded companies that are committed to producing nutritious food. They take the bounty of the first group and prepare it the way I would, if I had the time and expertise to do it all myself."

"That's who we like to buy from," Janice said. "When you read the labels on those products, you can see that they never compromise our health for the sake of convenience or sales."

"That's right," Fowler said. "But then there's the third group. And it's this group that makes way too many products that *do* compromise our health for the sake of our gotta-have-it-now, make-it-huge and make-it-tasty modern lifestyle."

"Because of the demands of our lifestyle," Janice said, "a lot of those companies take the wholesome natural food of the first group, and flip it around into burgers and fries and chips and doughnuts and candy and sodas, and anything else you can think of that's processed with added fat and sugar and chemicals whose names no one can pronounce."

"And those products are everywhere," Fowler said. "Even if you wanted, you couldn't ignore them. They're in our faces no matter where we are. In our homes. At work. In our grocery stores and convenience stores and drugstores and gas stations. Even strategically placed around our kids' schools." He shook his head.

"And *that*'s the problem. Because they're everywhere, they have become who we are. They define our modern lifestyle. So much so that we've come to believe that we *need* them. That our lives are even better because of them. But our lives *aren't* better, not when our weight continues to rise and our health continues to suffer."

"But what else is there?" Karen asked. "That kind of food is everywhere. And I have to say, it is fast and cheap and tasty and convenient."

"You're right," Fowler said. "It's all of that, we can't deny it. But I've turned the tables on that kind of food. With the right knowledge, I've become the one in control. I'm now the boss."

"You have the willpower to say no," Karen said.

Fowler shook his head. "If I was able to fit my willpower

into a thimble, there'd still be room left over for my thumb. No. That's not it."

"No one's willpower is strong enough to resist the pull of today's advertising powerhouses," Janice said. "Getting you to eat that type of food is a multi-billion-dollar business in itself. Those advertisers hire the greatest scientists and sharpest minds money can buy, and together they study us down to our genetic, primal urges. They know exactly how to get to us." She shook her head. "You can't fight that kind of bombardment with willpower."

Karen leaned back in her seat. "But that's what I've always done. Hang on for a while, resist the urge, eat my lettuce, then beat myself up for doing exactly what those advertisers want me to do. Go back to that kind of food—and fail."

"You and most of the country," Fowler said.

"Then what *can* I do?" Karen asked.

"Well, the one thing you *can't* do is passively try to resist them," Fowler said. "And you don't want to. That type of food *is* a part of our culture. A huge part. And because of that it'll always be a part of our lives. What you've got to do is take away its strength. Take back control. Karen, it is a war— for our children's health and our own. And to fight this war, like any other, you've got to be armed and ready. Armed with knowledge—and ready to make choices."

—⁊—

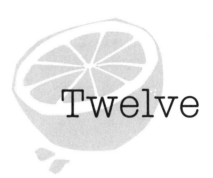

# Twelve

It was just past noon when Janice opened the front door. Fowler was right behind her. They both wore huge smiles for Karen.

Karen's first words, though, were, "I couldn't lie to him! I just don't know what he expects me to do! He practically forces me to leave, then makes it worse because I come here, the only place I can go!"

Janice's smile disappeared. For a moment she seemed to also be at a loss for words, then she simply said, "Come on in," and backed her chair deeper into the house, watchful for anyone who might be passing by. Fowler too, grimaced and shook his head at Karen's predicament. Then he turned his attention to Gabe, greeting him with an enthusiastic "Hey there, little man!" The baby gave him a series of gurgles and babbles in return. Fowler lifted him into his arms.

Karen closed the door behind her. She knew Gary's

refusal to accept her friendship with Fowler and Janice disturbed them. It had affected her too, but in a different way.

Staying home, doing as Gary wished, had at first seemed easier than coming here. It was effortless. And it carried the built-in rationalization that it was what Gary wanted. But even more than that, she knew, it was also that staying away from the Power of One Good Habit, not learning what Fowler knew, not failing at another diet, no matter what Fowler called it, seemed easier.

But she'd told herself no. She was going to continue through the door they'd opened, continue pushing forward.

Fowler gestured the two women toward the kitchen, saying softly to Karen, "We're really glad you came. I know this is hard for you."

The moment Janice steered herself through the kitchen doorway, though, she turned her chair around, looked up at Karen and said, "We don't have to do this, you know. You can be here—just to be here. Try it that way. We can have lunch without talking about losing weight."

"No!" Karen said. "I made up my mind. I want you to teach me what you know." *And I'll worry about Gary later*, she thought. She took the notebook Janice had given her from Gabe's diaper bag and opened it to the first page. On it, in large letters, she'd written, "The first step to the Power of One Good Habit is finding the *courage* to want to *learn*."

Fowler leaned over and read what she wrote. "Good," he said. "That's step one. And step two is to learn *what* there is to learn. And the best place to begin that is behind the counter."

"Then that's where I want to be," Karen said. She took Gabe from Fowler's arms and buckled him into the baby seat, releasing the snaps at the neck of his blue and yellow bodysuit. Janice switched on the radio and parked herself at the table next to him. One of her magazines filled with mathematical puzzles sat on the table. For now though, Janice left it untouched. Instead, she reached for Gabe's foot and tickled it. Gabe kicked out his legs, giving Janice an excited squeal, then grabbed his toes and tried to bring them to his mouth. Janice laughed lightly. Courage stretched out on the floor beside Janice's wheelchair.

Karen took out a set of colored rings from her bag and placed them within Gabe's reach. "I expect him to be asleep soon," she said to Janice. "He ate just before we left home, so now is his nap time."

"Should I leave him alone, then?" Janice asked.

"Not at all. Don't worry about him. He'll decide what he wants to do, won't you?" she asked the baby. She noisily buzzed his cheek with kisses, and confessed, laughingly, to Janice, "I could just eat him up!" Then she stepped over to the food-preparation area.

Fowler had poured three glasses of water and was now adding a slice of lemon to each. He handed one of the glasses to Karen, and bringing another to Janice, said over his shoulder, "I'm hungry . . . "

"Me too!" Karen chimed in.

"Good," Fowler said, stepping back behind the counter again. "Because what I have planned for lunch is a veal roll with spinach and cheese, long-grain brown rice with a combination of broccoli, cauliflower and carrots on the side and, of course, a green salad." He grinned. "What do you think? Will that do the trick?"

"Boy, will that ever!" Karen laughed. "My usual lunch is a burger or a deli sandwich, or a submarine with a bag of chips and a soda. Anything quick. I don't have time to fuss, especially if I'm working."

"Well, we'll see what this so-called fuss is," Fowler replied. "Ready to start?"

"You bet. What do I do?"

"First, take out the container of cut-up veggies with dip that I keep in the fridge. That's my cooking snack. Keeps me going until I eat."

"Keeps him going during the rest of the day too," Janice said. "That and fruit." She had adjusted Gabe's baby seat so the two of them could watch Karen and Fowler.

Fowler just shrugged. "I like to eat."

Karen put the veggies on the counter, picked out a piece of cauliflower, dipped it into the dip, and ate it. "Tangy," she said to Fowler, reaching for a second one.

"That's why I eat them. Because they're good, and they're there." He grinned, then said, pointing to the cupboard next to the refrigerator, "Okay. Why don't you start with the brown rice, and I'll get the veal going?"

"Brown rice, coming up," Karen said. She took a swallow of her water, then opened the cupboard door. "Well, well! We have choices here. Which one do you want, the quick-cooking or the regular?"

Fowler, reaching into the refrigerator for the veal, looked at her and said, "They're both a snap to prepare, but since the veal's going to take time to make, and then bake, and we're in no hurry, today's a good day for the regular. I usually save the quick-cooking kind for my gotta-eat-now-'cause-I'm-busy meals."

"*Those* meals are the norm," Janice said, directing this comment to Gabe, gesturing with her hands as though expecting him to reply. The baby watched her every move, then, with his fingers spread wide, he shouted, "Ga ga ga ga ga!"

"Okay!" Janice said.

Fowler laughed. He put the veal on the counter and said to Karen, "It's true. Most days I'm just too busy for the luxury of spending an hour in the kitchen. But today we have company, so that makes it special."

"Thank you," Karen said, reaching for the box of rice. Fowler added, "The pots are under the counter, next to the stove. Take out one of the large ones and just follow the directions on the package. They're foolproof." Then he quickly added, "Oh, yeah, and we'll need enough rice to serve ten."

"Ten!"

Both Fowler and Janice laughed. Fowler said, "Whenever I cook something that can be stored in the fridge or the freezer, then reheated and enjoyed again, I make more than the amount I need at the moment. Usually preparing a meal for four, or a meal for fourteen, no matter what it is, takes virtually the same amount of time. And even if it does take a little longer, what I'm doing is banking my energy. And that's something I'll tell you about later. Right now, what I want to do is start at the very beginning."

"Okay," Karen said. "Brown rice for a party of ten, coming up." She took another sip of her water, and dipped a baby carrot into the dip and popped it into her mouth. Then, following the instructions on the box, she filled the pot with water, added the rice, and placed the pot on the stove with the burner turned to high.

In the meantime Fowler had opened the packages of veal and put all nine pieces onto a plate. He said, "Let me first say, and I'll keep saying this, that what I'm going to be teaching you is not a diet. Diets don't work. It doesn't matter if it's a low-carbohydrate diet or a lowfat diet or the cabbage soup diet. They don't work because they're unsustainable. And that's because to keep them going you need to rely on willpower, and, if you're anything like me, willpower is in short supply."

"That," Karen said, "is the one thing I already know— from sad experience." *And,* she thought, *if that's really true, then the Power of One Good Habit takes away the worst pressure of a diet—concentrating on keeping up your willpower, having your whole world turn into what you can't eat, living with those horrible thoughts of being good or bad, of feeling anxious and guilty, always guilty. I hate that!*

"The other thing I want to say," Fowler continued, "is that with all my explanations, even if *I* know the minute details of why certain things are the way they are, I won't go to that depth. I'll say only what's necessary. If you want, you can get more information later, because it's easily available. But for our purposes, yours and mine, I'm sticking only to the major points, the ones that matter, because you have a life and I get tired of hearing my own voice. Okay?"

"Sounds perfect to me."

"Good. So let's get started, with the meal *and* the Power of One Good Habit." Fowler opened the drawer next to him, took out two meat pounders, and said to Karen, "Do you want the wooden one or the brass one? I started out years ago with the wooden one, then bought the brass type because I thought it would work better. But the truth is, they both do an excellent job."

"In that case," Karen said with a smile, "I'll take the brass one, just because it's shiny."

"Then the shiny one's for you," Fowler said, handing it to Karen. "Okay, the first thing we need to do is pound the veal slightly to flatten and tenderize it. And we'll also cut off any fat we find. So, just put a piece of the veal between two sheets of cellophane, like this," he said, demonstrating, "and lightly pound away."

"You're talking to a pro," Karen said, pulling out a sheet of cellophane. "I've done this before. The restaurant I used to work at was an off-campus free-for-all. We called it the Zoo. The menu looked like an encyclopedia, and we all had to do a little of everything, in the dining room *and* the kitchen." She laughed. "There was no such thing there as a job title, just a job!"

Fowler watched as Karen expertly pounded the veal, then said, "Well, all right then! On to the Power of One Good Habit!"

Karen laughed again. She looked over the counter at Janice and Gabe. Gabe was holding onto Janice's finger.

"The first thing you need to know," Fowler said, working on a piece of veal, "is that there are three kinds of foods. Carbohydrates, proteins, and fat. And our bodies were designed to need all three. That's what God did, not me. And he didn't give us any options either! So if anyone tells you the way to lose weight and gain health is by eating little or no carbohydrates or protein or fat, they're wrong. Just wrong. Always remember, when it comes to losing weight and gaining health, anything that doesn't sound like good common sense, anything that isn't *simple* sense, is usually *nonsense*. Got it?"

"Got it." Karen placed the flattened piece of veal onto a plate and put the next piece between sheets of cellophane.

"Okay. So our carbohydrates, or carbs, come from three kinds of foods. The starchy foods like bread, rice, pasta and potatoes—"

"The ones we're not supposed to eat," Karen said automatically, glancing at Fowler.

Janice laughed.

Fowler, shaking his meat pounder at Karen, said, "That's *exactly* what I mean! Do you hear yourself? You've been brainwashed by all those low-carb diet gurus. Think about it. If those diets really worked, the whole country would be thin by now."

Janice said, "Every few years, as each new low-carb diet comes along, we think low-carb dieting is the newest and greatest way to lose weight. But the truth is, low-carb diets have been coming and going for over a hundred years, and in all that time they've never worked. And that's because nutritionally, they make no sense." She held up one finger at a time, saying, "One, they're unhealthy. Two, they have side effects no one wants. And three, even if they do result in some weight loss, that loss is temporary, because no one can sustain that ridiculous way of eating for very long."

"I know that," Karen said, shaking her head. "I really do. I not only know it in my brain, but in my gut, 'cause I've been there. And still, when I get desperate enough, I think that's the way to go. Low-carbing. Because that's all I hear about."

"The power of mass marketing," Janice said, talking now to Gabe. "Sell an idea often enough, and it becomes truth."

"Okay," Fowler said, turning back to the veal. "Enough time wasted on nonsense! We need to eat carbs. That's not an opinion. It's a scientific given. And there are three basic types of carbs. First there's the starchy ones, like bread and potatoes and rice and pasta. Second are all the fruits and vegetables. And third is sugar in all its forms. They're all carbs. And

71

carbs are used by the body like—well, like the way my old clunker out there uses gas. It's our fuel."

Karen, placing another piece of veal between two sheets of cellophane, repeated the three categories to herself.

"Proteins, on the other hand," Fowler continued, also reaching for another piece of veal, "are basically everything that comes from a source that at one time or another breathed, and from certain plants. So that includes all animals, birds and fish, along with all their by-products. And also legumes, seeds and nuts."

"So proteins are meat and poultry, and dairy products and eggs?" Karen asked, turning to Fowler.

"Exactly. If you can trace the food's source back to something that used to breathe, plus those plant exceptions, it's most likely protein. And protein, if we go back to my clunker, is like me, that old car's mechanic. It does all the body's fixing and adjusting and maintaining." He reached for the final piece of veal.

"And the last type of food," he said, "is fat. And fat is anything that's greasy, like butter and oil and margarine and lard and shortening—and this," he said, picking up a strip of fat he'd trimmed from the veal. "And fat, just like carbs, can also be separated into three major types—"

Janice said, "You can call the fat categories the good, the bad and the ugly."

"That you can," Fowler agreed. "Basically, the good fat is called unsaturated fat, and that fat comes from foods like nuts and salmon, and oils like olive and canola. While the bad fat, on the other hand, is saturated fat. And that fat comes mostly from animals and their by-products, like beef, pork, poultry and eggs and dairy products. And the last one, the ugly fat, is manufactured. That one's called trans fat. And trans fat is found in most shortenings and margarines and cookies and crackers, and in just about every snack food that needs to last for months or years on a shelf."

"It was made for that purpose," Janice said. "To not break down over time."

Karen nodded at Janice. She could see that Gabe was slowing down. She gave him about five minutes before he closed his eyes.

"And fats," Fowler continued, "especially the good fats, are key to our health and weight. Not only do they make our food tastier and help us feel more satisfied when we eat, but if we go back to my old car again, they also act like all the different doohickeys and fluids that the car needs. Fat helps keep us lubricated and pliable and running trouble-free."

He finished flattening the last piece of veal, then opened a drawer and took out a box of wax paper. He pulled off two good-sized sheets and spread them on the counter, saying, "So. Like I said before, to be healthy, we need all three types of food—carbs, proteins and fat. But when it comes to fat, our modern culture has gone way overboard, so with fat we need to—"

"Here we go," Karen said, placing her meat pounder into the sink and washing her hands. "This is where we start to count. And this is where I always—"

But Fowler cut her off. "I said there'll be no counting of *anything* on my watch! No numbers. Not for anything. Life is complicated enough. Now write down what I'm going to tell you." He too stepped up to the sink and washed his hands.

The pot of rice had begun to boil. Karen lowered the heat and covered the pot, then reached for her notebook.

"Okay," Fowler said, drying his hands. "The enemy is out there—"

"All those food companies," Karen said.

"No! It's not the food companies that are the enemy. They're just answering the call, giving us what we ask for. The enemy is our modern culture. *That's* where the problem begins."

"It *is* that, isn't it?" Karen said, nodding slowly. She picked up her pen.

Fowler hung the towel over his shoulder and said, "One of the biggest weapons the enemy is using to harm us is

73

excess fat. Not just fat, because as I said, we all need fat, but *excess* fat. And that's what I want you to write."

Karen wrote this down and underlined it, then looked at Fowler.

"So our first line of attack," Fowler continued, "our first major counterstrike against the enemy, our first habit, is to reduce the amount of fat we eat—to as low a level as possible. And that's it. There's no counting of calories or fat grams or anything else. The number you're looking for isn't a number at all. It's simply, *as low as possible.* And this isn't some sort of rule or law. There's nothing firm about it. In some cases, as low as possible is zero, and at other times it's whatever it turns out to be. And that's just the way it is—because this is real life and not a diet."

"As low in fat as possible," Karen repeated. "But how do I go about—"

"In practically every situation," Fowler said, reaching for a slice of red pepper and spooning it through the dip, "there are only a few key ways to lower fat. Only a handful. And they're all simple. And as we get to them, I'll show you every one." He popped the red pepper into his mouth.

Janice said, "And once you know the key ways to lower fat, and see how easy they are, you'll be amazed at how fast this new habit gets absorbed into your life."

―

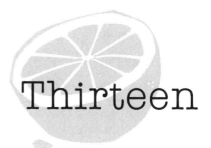

# Thirteen

"So we're on a hunt for fat," Karen said.

"That's exactly right," Fowler replied. "Always remember, this is war! And one of the enemy's most dangerous weapons is excess fat. Excess fat is his land mines, his tanks, his cruise missiles. And to defeat the enemy, you've got to eliminate his weapons. So the mission is to search out and destroy all that excess fat!"

Karen's brows were knitted in worry. "I know it seems easy when you say it. Find the fat and get rid of it. But in practice it'll be—"

"It'll be as easy as it sounds!" Fowler looked Karen in the eyes. "Listen to me. In some situations you'll be able to eliminate all the fat, without any effort. And in other situations, you won't. It's as simple as that. You do what you can, then move on with your life—without worry, without guilt. Just move forward."

He went to the refrigerator and took out two containers

of cheese, then took two packages of chopped spinach from the freezer. He popped the spinach into the microwave to thaw and held up the containers of cheese. "Look, I've made a choice with the cheese. I could have bought the kind that's high in fat or the kind that's low in fat. And I chose the low-fat, both for the feta and the cottage cheese. So where's the difficulty there?"

"There was none."

"Right! And the veal was a choice too. I could have taken anything off the shelf, but I chose a meat that's low in fat. And the visible fat that it did have, I removed. So I lowered the amount of fat even more. And," Fowler continued, spraying a baking dish with oil from a pump sprayer, "to oil the baking dish I'm using a sprayer instead of just pouring the oil from the bottle, so I'm using as little oil as possible, which is another way of reducing fat."

Karen, nodding and reaching for her notebook, said, "Okay, if I've got it right, there are two basic ways to get started: *choose* to reduce, and *limit* to reduce." She scribbled the words as she spoke them.

"That's exactly right. First, we choose foods that are as low in fat as possible, and then we see how we can limit the fat we do use, like the fat for cooking."

"The choosing part is easy," Janice said, adding, "Gabe's asleep. He just this second closed his eyes." She turned off the radio.

The three of them looked at Gabe for a moment, and then the microwave beeped. Fowler, taking out the spinach, said to Karen, "All right. We were talking about limiting fat. And like Janice said, the choosing part is easy. When I shop for food, I just steer clear of the artery-clogging bad fat, the animal fat. I just choose something else."

"What exactly do you stay away from?" Karen asked, picking up her pen again.

Fowler said, counting off on his fingers, "Whole and two-percent milk, all the regular fat-filled cheeses, all those thickly marbled meats, hot dogs and sausages of course, and even prime rib and some steaks. And don't for a second think I don't still enjoy meat and cheese. I don't eliminate them from my shopping trip, I simply go for the leaner cuts and the lower fat."

"But that's only part of it," Janice said, moving her wheelchair to the counter and reaching for the tray of cut vegetables. "The next step is in the cooking."

"You bet it is," Fowler said. "My biggest problem was that I used to be a fried-food type of guy. Whatever it was, I'd fry it. Just pour the oil in the pan, listen to the glub-glub-glub as it came out of the bottle, then throw whatever I was cooking into the oil and watch it soak up all that grease."

"The house used to stink!" Janice said.

Fowler smiled. "She's right. It *did* smell. But now I'm the Bake, Boil and Broil King. Unless there's no choice, I just don't fry. And when I do fry, I limit the amount of oil I use by spraying it on a pan instead of pouring it in."

Karen's head was bent over her journal. "Bake, boil and broil," she wrote.

"Then," Janice said, "there's limiting the ugly part of the good, the bad, and the ugly. The trans fat. I don't know why it's even legal!"

Fowler said, "A lot of the better manufacturers are getting rid of it. But it's still out there."

"So how do I limit trans fat?" Karen asked.

Fowler, reaching for a mixing bowl, looked at Janice, handing off the question to her.

"Well," Janice said. "A huge source of trans fat is in deep-fried restaurant food, like French fries. So as much as possible we should all avoid that. But I guess that's obvious. The rest of it's in packaged grocery products, and the easiest way to avoid trans fat there is to just read the package. If it says partially hydrogenated or trans fat on the label, put it back on the shelf." She smiled. "But you should also know that just because a product has a banner across the front of the package saying *Zero Grams of Trans Fat*, it doesn't necessarily mean it's one-hundred-percent trans fat-free."

"It doesn't?" Karen said. "How could it not? Isn't there a law about truth in advertising?"

"It's a quirk of the labeling laws. Some products—crackers or margarine, for example—might say *zero grams of trans fat per serving* on the label, but still have partially hydrogenated oil, which is trans fat, listed in the ingredients. So they still contain trans fat. They just have to have less than half a gram of the stuff *per serving* to be able to label it *zero grams of trans fat per serving*. The problem is, if you eat more than the listed serving size—and most people do—you're getting more trans fat than you should."

"That's ridiculous," Karen said. "I've seen those packages. They blare in big print *Zero Grams of Trans Fat*. And now you're telling me that if I read the list of ingredients, the small print, I might find that's not true?"

"For some items you will," Fowler said, breaking up the defrosted spinach into the mixing bowl. "But a lot of manufacturers have simply done the trans fat-to-saturated fat switcheroo, even some restaurants are doing it, switching from partially hydrogenated to fully hydrogenated. From the ugly to the bad. So they can say that it's zero grams of trans fat—but big deal! It's still the bad, saturated fat." He opened the container of cottage cheese and added it to the spinach.

Karen was shaking her head.

Janice said, "It's all listed on the nutrition label and in the ingredients list. Saturated fat *and* trans fat. We just have to be conscious about reading both, because those fats really aren't good for us."

"Okay," Karen said determinedly, more to herself than Janice or Fowler. "I have to start looking at the nutrition labels, and even the ingredients list, and start staying away from both saturated and trans fats. The bad and ugly. Because neither of them is doing me or Gary or Gabe any good." She made a flurry of notes on her pad.

Janice was nodding. Fowler, though, began to smile, as if he was holding back a secret. He began crumbling the feta cheese, adding it to the cottage cheese and the spinach.

"What? What is it? Why are you smiling?" Karen asked him, looking up from her pad.

Fowler said to Janice. "Now I have to tell her how to add back fat." Janice laughed.

Karen's eyes widened. "Add back fat? After you just showed me how to get rid of it? Why would you want to do that?"

Janice said, "The fat we add back is the good fat, the unsaturated fat, because it's so beneficial. The only thing is, we add it back in small, controlled amounts."

"Okay, now I'm really confused."

Fowler, with a wooden spoon in his hand, said, "Actually, it's simple. What's confusing is the way it's been told to us by all the professionals out there, the scientists and nutritionists and doctors. Think about it. First they said, the answer to losing weight was just to eat lowfat—"

"I remember that!" Karen interrupted. "And I jumped all over it, eating as much as I liked of whatever said lowfat or fat-free, especially all those fat-free snacks. And my weight ballooned!"

"A lot of people got caught up in that mistake," Janice said. "All the diet industry did was get rid of the fat and replace it with sugar. Of course people gained weight. Weight gain is about calories, not just fat."

"It was after that," Fowler said, mixing the ingredients in his bowl, "that the scientific community began to realize that not all fats are the same."

"You mean not all fat is bad?" Karen asked.

"That's right," Fowler said. "The ones Janice talked about before—good, bad, and ugly. Unsaturated, saturated, and trans fat. So now, once they figured out how these different types of fats affected our health, the professionals said, 'Okay, eat the right amount of the good fats—and don't eat the bad.' Just like that. I've read that sentence dozens of times. The trouble is, no one knows what that means. Not in real life, anyway. I mean, what are we supposed to do, go into a restaurant and ask for only the good fats and not the bad? It's just not practical."

Janice said, "The scientists who study these things and tell us what to do, they mean well, they just don't know how to explain what they're saying in a way that tells us how to apply it to real life. My father had to figure that out for himself."

Fowler turned to Karen. "The problem with saying 'Eat only limited amounts of good fat, but don't eat the bad,' is that two distinct steps have been combined into one. And when we try to do it that way, all in one step, we mess it up. Then, because we're really not sure what we're doing, we just ignore it, or stop thinking about good and bad fats altogether."

"It took my father years to figure out the right way to look at it," Janice said. "But once he figured it out, not only did it work easily, it also fit into his life the way he likes everything about the eight habits to fit in—in a way where he doesn't have to think about them."

"One day it just came to me," Fowler said. "All I had to do was divide that sentence into two separate steps. Easy steps. First, limit the bad fats, and then, once I had that covered, add back small amounts of the good, because we really need those good fats for our health. And suddenly it worked perfectly."

Karen said, "So you began by limiting all the excess fat . . . "

"Exactly. And what I saw when I focused on that, was that most of the excess fat I was eating was the bad fat, saturated fat."

"That's all the full-fat cheeses and whole milk and fatty meats you listed, right?" Karen said, glancing at her notes.

"That's right. And fat-laden fried foods and gravies and baked goods. It's really not a long list, but it was a *lot* of saturated fat. So that's how I began, by eliminating all the excess 'bad fats' from my life, in a way that I could live with, by either cutting them out or cutting them down, whatever was convenient for the situation. And I did that until it became second nature."

"Then he added step two," Janice said.

Fowler nodded. "Janice began to tell me—"

"Over and over," Janice interrupted.

Fowler laughed and reached for the platter of cut vegetables. "It's true, it took a while for it to sink in. But when I finally began to see all the benefits that the good fats can provide, I thought, Okay, I have all those bad fats under control, so the thing to do now is to add back some of the good fats—for what they can do for me." He tossed a baby carrot into his mouth.

"In limited amounts," Janice said, also reaching for the vegetable platter, "because those good fats still have calories."

Fowler nodded. "And that's what I did. I began to add back small amounts of the good fats into what I was eating. I mean, I consciously looked for them. And I can tell you that all it took was one blood test, a few months later, for me to see that I was on the right track. Because limiting the bad fat, and then adding back small amounts of the good, did wonders for my cholesterol."

"The good fat actually improves your HDL, your good cholesterol," Janice said. "And it fights the bad cholesterol. That's why it's so important. It also adds lubrication to our joints and elasticity to our arteries and veins. And in fact, new studies are now showing that the good fats, the unsaturated fats, also help prevent inflammatory diseases like arthritis and atherosclerosis—you know, clogging of the arteries."

"Really?" Karen said. "They're that good?"

"You bet," Fowler said.

"So what are the good fats?" Karen asked, her pen poised over her notepad once again. "If there's a list of the bad, then what's the list of the good?"

Fowler said, "It's a short list, so it's easy to remember. The good fats are in nuts and seeds, things like peanuts, almonds, sesame, and flax. Fish, too, like salmon and sardines. And unsaturated plant-based oils like olive, canola and peanut oil."

"And in avocados," Janice said. "And all those fats are excellent for us."

"More than excellent," Fowler said, "I can tell you from experience that they're essential. But they still have calories, just like any other kind of fat. So while we add them back into our oil tanks for their benefits, we also don't want the tank to overflow. So, for example, with almonds, one of my favorite snacks, I'll have ten or so at a time, not fifty. Or twenty or so peanuts instead of twenty *handfuls*. And with the oil, it's still from the pump sprayer and not just poured from the bottle."

"Okay," Karen said, taking a deep breath. "I think I get it. First, step one, take out the excess fat in my life by choosing foods that are low in fat, and by limiting the amount of overall fat that I use. And I can do this both in my home and when I eat out, because it's just a matter of making the right choice. And since a lot of the excess fat is bad fat—"

"And ugly," Janice interrupted. "Most snacks foods are still pumped full of trans fat."

"Okay, it's getting clearer now," Karen said. "I limit the bad and the ugly, then, at home, or whenever I can, I add back small amounts of the good for my health."

"That's exactly it," Fowler said. "And that, in a healthy nutshell, is the first habit. Find the fats—and know the good, the bad, and the ugly. Choose foods that are as low in fat as possible, and then add back limited amounts of the good fats. And no matter the outcome, our mission is always a total success—because we do what we can without any sacrifice or struggle, then move on with our lives."

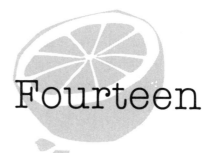

# Fourteen

"So it's really that easy," Karen said. "Keep what I eat as low in fat as possible, to keep the bad fats down, then add back a few good fats here and there. And there's no counting."

Her voice, however, sounded doubtful. She knew that every diet she'd ever tried had always sounded this way at the beginning. Simple and infallible. And that whoever was selling the diet, whether it was a friend or a professional pitchman, always sounded just like Fowler was sounding now, as though having her accept the diet was the most important thing in the world. *But,* she thought, *so far this one does sound simple, doesn't it?*

Fowler ignored Karen's tone. "You don't count anything. Ever. You go for as low in fat as possible, whatever that turns out to be. Keep an eye out for adding back some of the good fats when you can. And then move on."

"But what about the rest?" Karen said, glancing at her

notes. "You said that to be healthy we need all three types of food—carbs, proteins, and fat."

"That's coming," Fowler replied. "Let's get on with the meal first."

At this Karen first dipped her head. Then, as an after-thought, she saluted. Fowler returned the salute with a quick, full-bodied laugh. He told Karen to turn on the oven, and went back to the veal. He placed the flattened pieces of veal on the wax paper, laying them out so that each piece over-lapped the other by about half an inch. Then he gave the overlap a quick pound to join the pieces together. After spic-ing the veal, he pointed at the pot of rice on the stove and asked Karen, "What type of food is that?"

"It's one of the starchy foods. So it's a carb."

"Right. And what about the cheese in the mixing bowl?"

"That came from an animal, so it's a protein."

"She's got it," Fowler said to Janice.

"She does," Janice agreed.

Fowler spiced the cheese and spinach combination with a dash of salt and freshly ground pepper, gave it another quick mix, then spread it in a thin layer over the veal. Then he gen-tly lifted one side of the wax paper and began to roll the veal over itself without letting the wax paper roll with it.

Karen, nodding her head in admiration, said, "You've got that technique down pat."

"Learned it from a cooking show," Fowler said.

"He records them," Janice said. "Cooking shows and gar-dening shows."

Fowler laughed. "Movies, too! The older the better. Espe-cially the westerns!"

"When he grows up he wants to be John Wayne," Janice said.

When the veal was completely rolled, Fowler placed it on the baking dish and put the dish into the preheated oven. "There, I'm done. And in no time at all this'll be at least *ten* meals!" He turned to Karen, "I just thought of another one.

Do you remember what I did with the egg yolks this morning, when I was making the French toast?"

"I sure do. You threw most of them in the garbage."

"So what was I doing?"

"You . . . were eliminating fat."

"Right. And what type of fat?"

"Animal fat, so it's saturated fat, the bad fat."

"That's it!" Fowler said. Then in a more serious tone, he added, "Karen, I told you there are only a handful of key ways to search out and destroy fat, and now you know four of the best. And if you use only those, replace as many products as possible with their lowfat equivalents. Use lean cuts of meat and poultry and remove all the apparent fat. Use limited numbers of egg yolks only if you need your eggs to look yellow. And use a pump sprayer when you need to oil your pans, you'll be miles ahead of where you are now. Miles!"

Though Karen smiled and nodded, she still knew it all seemed too easy. *But I am impressed,* she thought, *because I will try those ideas. And I wasn't planning on trying anything. All I wanted was to understand how the Power of One Good Habit worked.*

Fowler said, "What you're going to find is that after a while, after you've been hunting and destroying fat for a few months, you'll begin to lose your taste for it."

"Lose my taste for fat?" Karen laughed. "That's hard to believe!"

"You will. Six months from now, after becoming a non-fried-foods kind of person, you might go into a restaurant and splurge on some extra-crispy fried chicken. And you'll see, you won't like the feel of it in your throat or on the top of your mouth. It might even upset your stomach. The body loses the urge for it."

Karen shook her head, amazed. "I had no idea that could happen."

Janice said, "I don't know why, but it's true."

"You can count on it," Fowler said. "It happened to both

of us." He was still smiling at Karen's surprise. "Okay, back to the meal. What else was on the menu?"

"The rest of the menu," Karen repeated. "Let's see. Oh yes, broccoli, cauliflower and carrots, and a green salad." Then she added, "You know, about now, if I was alone and the cooking was being done because it had to be done, and not because I was having a good time, I'd be getting pretty tired of it." She leaned against the counter. "Actually, to be honest, at this point I doubt if I'd want to do anything else— not prepare the broccoli or cauliflower, or peel any carrots, or clean the lettuce." She shook her head. "It's what Gary always says. It's my lazy streak."

"Wait a minute!" Fowler objected at once. "There's a huge difference between being lazy and being tired. Or needing a break. Or getting a hand once in a while. You're a mother and a wife and you work outside the home. And in today's world we don't have to work in the fields to get tired. Just sitting at a desk and handling our responsibilities is work enough. Even if you were a stay-at-home mom, handling your responsibilities in the house *and* in your relationships can be more than enough. And if sometimes you do feel lazy, well, I'll raise your lazy with two of my own, because we've all got a lazy streak in us."

Karen looked grateful at Fowler's explanation. *You're right,* she thought. *I'm not a lazy person, just sometimes tired. And if there are times when I decide to feel lazy, then that's all right too!*

Fowler said, "I'm going to show you two ways to get around being tired. And if you want to call it lazy, then we'll call it lazy. A very, very positive lazy."

He went over to the freezer. "First, here's our broccoli, cauliflower and carrots." He took out a bag of California blend broccoli, cauliflower and carrots, poured it into a pot, filled the pot with about an inch of water, and put it on to boil. "There. Done. One minute, maybe less. Now the salad." He went to the refrigerator, took out a bag of store-bought pre-washed greens, opened the bag, and poured them into a bowl. Then he added a small handful of crushed almonds to the salad and asked, "What am I doing?"

Karen said, "You're adding back good fat!"

"Right," Fowler said. Next he added a dozen cherry tomatoes to the crushed almonds, then on top of it all, poured a couple of tablespoons of lowfat salad dressing. "There's the salad," he said. "And it's a beaut. And all it took was another minute or two."

Karen was smiling. *You got me,* she thought.

Fowler turned to her and said, "Karen, the Power of One Good Habit is real life, not playing house. Not playing diet. Not playing at anything. If there's something out there that's nutritious and quick to prepare and fits into the concept of any of the habits, go for it! We're not here to be martyrs or masochists."

Janice said excitedly, "Look at Gabe. He's still fast asleep, but he's shaking his hands. He must be having a dream!"

Karen stepped to the table. She unbuckled the baby from the baby seat and lifted him into her arms, pressing her head next to his. Gabe continued to sleep. Karen said to Janice, "Would you like to hold him?"

"Can I? Oh yes! I was going to ask, I just didn't know if that was okay, I mean, to ask to hold someone else's baby."

"It's perfectly all right," Karen said, stepping over to Janice. "People always want to hold babies." She placed Gabe on Janice's lap, telling her how to place her arms.

"It's so wonderful," Janice said, staring at Gabe, her eyes moist. "It's just so wonderful. A new life. A perfect life. So innocent."

Karen glanced at Fowler. His eyes too were moist. He smiled at Karen, then turned away. He checked the rice. Turned off the burner. Then looked in the oven. "Five more minutes," he said to no one in particular.

For the next few minutes Karen and Fowler both watched Janice hold the baby. She was rocking him slightly, though she hadn't been told to do this.

"He'll probably sleep through lunch," Karen said. "And

I'm really looking forward to the day when he begins to sleep through the night."

"When will he begin to talk?" Janice asked, never taking her eyes off Gabe.

"The books say he'll start talking somewhere between eighteen months and two years."

"You began early," Fowler said to Janice. "At just over a year I started to make out combinations of words. Then a few weeks later you got your PhD . . . Well, okay, maybe not, but it seemed like that!" He checked the oven again, and this time said, "Okay. Time to eat." He put on a pair of oven mitts and took out the veal.

Janice said to Gabe, "It's time for you to go back into your baby seat." She leaned to him and touched the top of his head with her lips, then looked up at Karen.

Karen placed Gabe back into the baby seat. Janice, meanwhile, steered her wheelchair out of the kitchen, saying, "I'll be back in two minutes." Courage followed her.

Karen stepped into the cooking area.

Fowler whispered to her, "Thank you."

Karen, knowing exactly what Fowler meant, said, "She's so sweet, so gentle . . . "

Fowler took a deep breath. Then, clearing his throat, he said, "You were talking about your lazy streak, and I was telling you about mine. So now I want you to watch, because I'm going to teach you another way to blow that term *lazy* off the map!"

He took three plates from one cupboard, then pulled seven plastic containers out of another. He lined the containers in a row and, after slicing the veal into ten equal portions, placed one portion into each of the containers, along with a good serving of the brown rice and a hefty helping of the broccoli, cauliflower and carrots. Then he sealed the containers and said, touching each container after the other, "This is for your lunch tomorrow. And this is your dinner on Wednesday. And this one is a late-night snack in July. And this is your breakfast sometime in September."

"Yuck."

"Hey, that's good food! Just 'cause it's called breakfast, doesn't mean it has to abide by any rules." He grinned. "And the last three are for whenever you want." Then he took Karen by the elbow, led her to the freezer, opened the door and said, "Look in here. All of these, all fifteen or twenty different meals and snacks, were made when the making was good. When the energy level was high. Or just when I had to cook something, anything, and out of habit made more than I needed and stored the rest here, in my energy bank, for those days or nights or mornings when the only thing on my mind is to throw something into the microwave and drop my butt into a chair."

Janice, steering her wheelchair back into the kitchen, said, "I don't think you can call someone lazy who's prepared for their tired times. A more correct term would be ingenious."

"I don't know about that," Fowler said, shrugging. "All I know is that the freezer, for me, is just another tool. One that fits my style. And nothing more. It may not work for everyone." He turned to Karen. "Like everything else about the Power of One Good Habit, you have to assess it for yourself. Make sure it makes life *easier* for you, not harder. If making all your meals on the spot works best for you, then that's the way to go. The key is always preparation, having the ingredients on hand for nutritious meals that can be made in one or five or fifteen minutes."

He stacked the seven containers of food and put them aside, saying, "Okay, now you know that the first habit is to choose foods that are as low in fat as possible, and then to add back small amounts of the good fats for your health. All by making thoughtful choices. And to do it without any sacrifice or struggle, without any anxious or guilty feelings. And especially without letting this habit intrude into your life. So now let's see how all three types of food look when they're actually on our plates."

He put the remaining three portions of veal onto the

three plates. Then he added the brown rice and a serving of the broccoli, cauliflower and carrots to each. In a separate bowl, he heaped a hefty portion of the salad. "Okay," he said, "if you look at what we have, you'll see that one part of the plate has the veal and cheese . . . "

"The protein," Karen said.

"Right. And," Fowler said, holding out his hand, "you can also see that the portion size for the protein is no bigger than my palm."

"I taught him that," Janice said.

"That and much more," Fowler added, smiling at his daughter. Then he pointed at the rice on the plate and said to Karen, "What's this?"

"That's the carbs?"

"Exactly, the carbs. And here," he said, holding out his hand and closing it, "you can see that the portion is no bigger than my fist. Another good indicator."

"Palm for the protein, and fist for the carbs," Karen repeated. She quickly jotted that into her notebook.

"Exactly," Fowler answered. "And for the ever-important vegetables, they can cover the rest of the plate. And the salad is in a bowl by itself, a bowl that I like to see overflowing. And that's it. That's how our plates look. As simple as that."

"And the fat," Karen said, "because of the concept of search and destroy, of making it as low in fat as possible, is also where it's supposed to be. And there was no counting. Not of anything."

"It all begins with taking care of the fat," Fowler said.

Karen said, "Find the fat and eliminate it, then find places to sneak back in a bit of the good fats."

"That's what this habit is all about," Fowler said, grinning. And that's all you have to remember."

"It *is* simple, isn't it?" Karen said.

―↗―

90

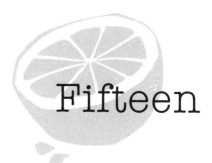

# Fifteen

For the next three days Karen was at work, so she had no opportunity to visit Janice and Fowler. The weekend was spent quietly, with Gary mostly watching sports on television. In the past week his only mention of Janice and Fowler had been a quick aside about "those nuts in the woods."

Though she didn't see Fowler and Janice, Karen telephoned. She was overjoyed to find that they were as happy to hear from her as she was to speak to them. She arranged to go to their house first thing Monday, and the moment Gary left for work that morning she bundled Gabe into his stroller.

She hadn't done anything about the first habit during the past five days except think about it. Go over and over in her mind the things Fowler had so far explained. Now she whispered, "I'm an idiot!" and thought, *What he's told me so far is ridiculously easy. There's not even any effort involved. It's all just a matter of choices. Of letting the smallest amount of courage*

*move me forward a step. Just a single step. And then letting an-
other jolt of courage, another tiny amount, move me forward the
next small step. That's all he asked. And still I haven't been able
to start it! A pound a week, that's all he wants. Week after week.
Month after month . . .*

She stopped in mid-stride. *Wait a minute! What I'm doing
is filling my brain with doubts by looking at that end of it, at how
long it's going to take, when I ought to be looking at it from this
side. The now. Today. Looking only at the first step Fowler talked
about. Only that. I'm basing beginning the Power of One Good
Habit on what I don't know instead of what I do know!*

She knew that there was a key there somewhere, her key
to making the habits work. *Today. That's the key! Small steps—
and today. Now!* But with this thought she winced, feeling the
old familiar mix of fear and dread rise up from the knot in
her gut. *Courage. It always keeps coming back to that. That tiny
amount of courage. That first step: courage. The courage I need to
get me to do what has to be done—today. Without thinking about
tomorrow. And then tomorrow will just be another today. And all
of it without the old diet mentality.*

She reached into her tote bag and took out her notebook.
Kneeling next to Gabe, she wrote: "The enemy is out there.
And it's what's making me fat. It's not my fault—no matter
what Gary thinks! But I can defeat the enemy. Fowler's
proven that by doing it. And the weapons I need to defeat
the enemy are courage and knowledge."

She read this through and underlined *courage* and *knowledge*, then wrote: "Knowledge can be acquired, I see that now.
I can learn to do this. There's nothing difficult about what
Fowler's telling me. But courage, that's something else altogether. I don't know where courage comes from. I never
have."

\* \* \*

Janice greeted Karen and Gabe with another warm welcome.
This time though, she said, "Why don't we go into the den

until my father wakes up? That way we can talk without disturbing him."

Janice led the way, closing the door after Karen, motioning her to an easy chair alongside one of the desks where the computer was switched on. "I was working," she explained, stopping her chair in front of the desk. She reached out to touch Gabe. This morning he had no response for Janice.

"He had the sniffles most of the night, poor thing," Karen said, "so he'll probably spend the day catching up on his sleep." She smoothed Gabe's hair, adjusting him in her arms, positioning herself in the chair so she could see what Janice was doing. The computer screen was filled with text. She began to read the first line, bumping into unfamiliar words: Monocultures. Biodiversity and Transgenic.

Janice said, "I'm part of a team based in London that's researching the safety of genetically modified foods for use by the United Nations."

"London?"

Janice nodded. "I do a lot of work over the Internet."

"Is this your job?" Karen asked, looking at the screen once more.

"No. It's a nonprofit group, so there's no salary. But I'm glad to do it. I've been offered a position with another think-tank, though—several, actually—but of course it's impossible for me to work."

"Why?"

For a moment Janice only stared at Karen. Then she said, "Because I can't leave this house, can't let myself be seen. Because people are . . . shocked." She paused for a moment, then in a lowered voice added, "I can only imagine how my father felt when he first saw me. And my mother . . . " She let the word *mother* fade, before saying, "For a long time it was hard on him, having to deal with someone like me, a one-in-a-million mistake with complication after complication."

Karen reached out and touched Janice's hand, holding it for a moment without speaking.

"Fortunately, things changed," Janice said, her voice resuming its usual tone.

"Changed?" Karen said. "Because of the Power of One Good Habit?"

Janice nodded. "It's impossible to tell you how much those eight core habits turned my father's life around. And because they changed *his* life, they changed *mine*, too."

Karen thought of the bottle of whiskey and the package of cigarettes on the wall of Fowler's restaurant, the pair of trousers mounted like a trophy, and realized they represented the most significant successes of Fowler's life. He'd found the Power of One Good Habit, opened its door, and he and Janice stepped through it into a new world. *If only the same could happen to me and Gary.* She suddenly said, "Tell me about your father," then quickly added, "if that's all right. I mean . . . I don't mean to pry."

Janice smiled. "Of course it's all right." Then she said firmly, "I love him," adding, "Just like everyone else, he had his problems—he still does. And one of those problems is me, I guess. And at first he handled those problems the way a lot of people do, by using crutches—food, alcohol, cigarettes—to get him through the day. Using them to comfort himself. And like a lot of people, he didn't notice or care what he was doing until his escapes"—she put quotation marks around the word with her fingers—"became his largest problems. They took over his life. When he first decided to do something about it all, he weighed over three hundred pounds."

"Really!" Karen said. "But how did he start? I mean . . . what was . . . what did . . . ?" She searched for the right word.

Janice said, "You mean, what was the spark? Besides his mirror, that is?"

Before she could answer her own question, the door opened and Fowler, sleep still in his eyes, peeked into the room. "I saw the stroller in the hall," he said. "Good morning."

"I guess he can tell you himself what the spark was,"

Janice said to Karen. She turned to Fowler. "Karen wants to know what spark, besides your mirror, got you to develop the eight habits."

Fowler stepped into the room. "Actually, the spark wasn't my mirror. All the *mirror* did was make me feel guilty and weak."

"Then what was the spark?" Karen asked.

Fowler sat down in an armchair opposite Karen and Janice. "It was anger. I was angry. Furious! At myself, at my size, at my food, at my mirror. At all of it. And I used that anger to begin my journey."

"And create the eight habits?" Karen asked.

"Eventually. But only after a thousand attempts, after a hundred useless diets that restricted what I ate. That put me on pills, or liquids, or limited amounts of carbs. All of them tied to willpower, and all designed to make me lose thirty pounds in thirty days, so I could gain back thirty-five a month later." He grinned.

Karen's expression, though, was somber. "I know you keep saying the Power of One Good Habit isn't a diet. But if it's not a diet, then what is it?" She shifted Gabe, suddenly aware of his weight. His pacifier dropped from his mouth and she put it back in.

Janice said, "I've thought about that. And I think what it is, is a map."

"A map?" Karen said.

"That's right. A nutritional road map. Pointing the way from here to the city of Health." Janice paused, then added, "But it's even more than that. It's a new way of thinking. It's tomorrow, beginning now. In five or ten or twenty years, the Power of One Good Habit will be the nutritional road map the nation will be using—because it's based not only on science, but also on real life and good common sense. People won't let the enemy win this war—because they can't afford to, for their health's sake. So they'll ultimately dictate the way things are going to be, for themselves and their children, and not the other way around. Not the way it is now."

Karen was nodding, thinking not only about what Janice had just said, but also about the entry she'd made in her journal on the way over. "If the first step to the Power of One Good Habit is just a tiny amount of courage, just enough to say to myself that I really want to lose weight and that I'll make the simple choices at hand, then why is it that even that small amount is so hard for me to find?"

Fowler, after reflecting on the question, said, "I think the short answer is fear. You're afraid. And you're afraid of two things. First, you're afraid of having to give up the foods you've grown to depend on. Your comfort foods. Whether it's ice cream or chocolate or pizza or anything else. Those foods have become extremely important to you, to your life. And, second, it's the old fear of failure. And those two fears work hand in hand."

"How?" Karen asked.

"Well," Fowler said. "Over the years we've been swayed by everything from word-of-mouth to slick, hour-long infomercials playing on our sense of guilt or shame, talking us into trying too many wonder diets, too many magic pills. And all we got for our efforts—our sincere efforts—was failure. Not only did we have to give up what we liked, and even needed—those comfort foods we'd grown up with—but we were also forced into complicated programs of calorie counting or fat gram counting or trying to keep straight in our heads or in little booklets which food we were allowed to eat with which other food and on what day and at what time of day. And on and on and on . . . ."

Karen nodded. "I know it all, too well."

"So do I," Fowler said. "And the problem is that in time, all that nonsense and intrusion into our real, everyday lives became too much, so we ultimately end it—end the diet—and end it in failure, even if we'd lost some weight. Because diets are not sustainable. And that made failure our only frame of reference when it came to losing weight, to dieting. And it was that reference we carried with us on our next attempt. But by now our minds were saying, 'No! I won't put myself through that again. The struggle's too hard. It's too painful, and not worth it. I won't set myself up for another failure!'"

Janice was watching Karen. "Sound familiar?"

"Oh, yeah."

Fowler nodded along with her. "Or else we *did* give it another try, did get lured into another irresistibly slick wonder diet. But by now the attempt was half-hearted, no matter what we said, even to ourselves. It was half-hearted on the inside, where it counts. Why? Because by now we *knew* we were going to fail. We were living with the diet mentality of pain and guilt and failure. We expected failure, and so, naturally, we did fail. And still do. *Always*. I know the cycle. I lived it over and over and over."

Janice asked gently, "Is that what you're afraid of now, Karen? That you're going to fail at losing weight with the Power of One Good Habit?

Karen nodded.

Fowler asked, "Even though you know that the eight habits are not a diet? That they accommodate life, become a part of it, don't interfere with it? And that with the eight habits there's no such thing as a food you aren't allowed to eat?"

For a moment Karen just gazed at Fowler, weighing his question, then she nodded again and in a resigned tone said, "I'm sorry. It just doesn't matter how you describe it. In my mind we're still talking about a diet, and I still need courage to attempt it. And you were exactly right when you said my lack of courage comes from fear. And exhaustion from that diet mentality. I'm tired of failing and my mind is screaming at me that I'm gonna fail again. That I'm only going to disappoint myself, and disappoint you, and, for the thousandth time, confirm Gary's opinion of me."

For a long moment no one spoke. Then Fowler said, "I know what you're feeling. I really do. Because I've been there. And I also know it's useless for me to try to talk you into changing those feelings. So I won't."

"You won't?" Karen repeated, suddenly disappointed. She turned to Janice, who also looked let down.

Fowler shook his head. Then, grinning, said, "What I will do is *prove* to you, right now, that the Power of One Good Habit is different. That it's not a diet. That there's no struggling with it. And that it can so completely fit into your life, you won't even know it's there."

He waited an instant before asking, "What did you do with the seven meals I gave you the last time you were here?"

Karen smiled sheepishly. "I ate them."

"When did you eat them?"

"I ate the first two on the same day you gave them to me. One for dinner, then the other after Gary went to bed."

Fowler said, "That's good."

"But I ate the same meal three times in one day, once for lunch with you, then again for dinner, then again for a late-night snack."

"So what? Your body doesn't care about that. All your body wants is for the meals you eat to be nutritious. And they were. When did you eat the rest?"

"You're going to laugh at me," Karen said.

Fowler's expression told her differently.

"I ate another for lunch at work the next day, warming it in the microwave. Then I had another for dinner, also at work, because I stayed late. Then I had another after Gary went to bed, around ten-thirty."

"Excellent!"

"You mean it?"

"Of course! You had three nutritious, lower-in-fat-than-usual meals in one day. That's great. What about the rest?"

"Gary ate them. I just heated them together and put them on a plate and told him it was from the deli, and he wolfed it down."

Fowler laughed. "Okay. Now I'm going to make my point. Prove that you can't fail with the eight habits." He paused, looked Karen in the eyes, then said, "No matter what else you did last week, you already broke the enemy's grip on you—because you had five meals that were nutritionally perfect. You struck perfection five times. With that, you had your first success. Advanced your health. You did it, Karen! You met the goal of the Power of One Good Habit!"

It took a moment for Karen to fully grasp what Fowler had just said. Then, with a wondering smile spreading across her face, she whispered, "I *have* advanced my health, haven't I?"

"Yes!"

"And advancing my health is the goal of the Power of One Good Habit?"

"Yes!"

"And part of advancing my health is losing weight?"

"Yes!"

Karen's eyes were wide, alight. "And it was because of those five meals. That's all it took. And it happened without me even realizing it."

"That's the way the habits are designed to work," Fowler said. "Without you even realizing it. They disappear *into* your life, instead of being an *intrusion* on it." He grinned. "What are you feeling now? At this exact moment?"

"I'm feeling that I want to eat more of those meals! Push myself even further ahead."

"Further ahead? Keep meeting the goal? Keep acquiring successes? Keep gaining health and losing weight?"

"Yes!"

"Well, that feeling is not accidental. That's the momentum created by the Power of One Good Habit. When you see how simple it is to know, for sure, that you've achieved a degree of health, then you want to push yourself even further."

"But it was so easy!" Karen said. "Almost *too* easy. All I did was eat."

"All you did was adjust to the circumstances at hand, and not fall into the all-or-nothing trap of the diet mentality. Those meals were there and you ate them. The Power of One Good Habit slipped into your life. And remember, all you know so far is the first habit. And even with that, you still don't know all I'm going to teach you. Imagine when you have all the knowledge inside you. All eight habits! Imagine having an infinite number of combinations to work with, to adjust to your life and personal circumstances!"

"I'll be able to use what I want of the habits then," Karen said. "Let *them* adjust to *me*. Fit *me*!" Gabe reached for his pacifier and pulled it from his mouth, throwing it to the floor. Karen made a movement to stand, but Fowler motioned for her to stay seated.

He stood and picked up the pacifier and handing it to Karen, said, "You're exactly right. And *that's* why you can't fail. Because once the knowledge is in you, once you understand each of the habits, you can then tailor each one to suit your life at every moment, no matter the situation. And then readjust it. And you'll still, always, be moving toward the goal."

"My goal is to lose weight!"

"No!" Fowler's voice was sharp. "Your goal is to gain health—*only* that—incrementally and continuously, for the rest of your life. If your weight is a health problem, then your weight will be reduced." He sat back in the armchair.

"It's that focus too that makes it different," Karen said. "Sort of puts it into a different light. The Power of One Good Habit isn't just for overweight people, it's for everyone."

"That's right. It's not a diet—and it's not specifically for overweight people. It's for anyone who cares about their health and the health of the people they love."

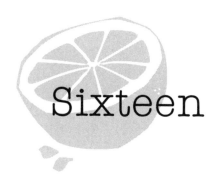

# Sixteen

"Then I want to learn more!" Karen said.

Janice, pointing at her computer screen, said, "I've still got a good hour's work here." She looked at Gabe and said softly, "He's closing his eyes."

"He needs to catch up on his sleep," Karen said, adding to Gabe, "Couldn't you have done this last night?" She looked at Janice. "I was up with him for hours. He's beginning to sleep through most of the night, thank goodness, but last night was just awful. At least I didn't have to go to work today. Poor Gary, when he left this morning he looked like he hadn't slept in a week."

Fowler said to Karen, "Why don't we go into the restaurant and have a coffee and talk? And when Janice is ready, we'll cook a Power of One Good Habit breakfast.

"Can Gabe stay here?" Janice asked. "My father can bring in the cradle."

"What do you think?" Fowler said to Karen.

"Sure. That would be fine."

Janice whispered to the baby, "You're going to stay with me!"

Fowler said. "Okay, then. I'll go get the cradle." He stood, mouthing the word *coffee?* to Janice. She nodded.

A few minutes later, Fowler had made coffee and brought one to Janice, then rejoined Karen at the kitchen table. Karen had her notebook open in front of her. She took a sip of her coffee and said, "You already gave me four simple ways to reduce fat, but a few minutes ago you said there was still more to the first habit."

"That's right, there is more." Fowler sipped his coffee, then said, "There's a basic rule to keep in mind about fat, and that is that fat is almost everywhere. So our first job is to find the fat. Think about it. You can only get rid of it after you've found it. So that's what I did. I first found the fat, and then I got rid of it. And that's how I created my *defatted* haven."

"Your what?" Karen asked.

Fowler, smiling, swept his hand to encompass the cooking area. "Come with me, and I'll show you what you don't see in my defatted haven." He stood, and Karen followed him around the counter to the refrigerator. Fowler opened the door and said, "Okay, what don't you see?"

Karen looked in, thought about it, then realized she had no idea what Fowler was talking about. "How can I tell you what I don't see?"

"Let me help," Fowler said. "The first thing you don't see is butter."

"That's right, there's no butter."

Fowler grinned. "No butter. No full fat mayo. No full fat cheeses. No full fat milk . . . In every case I found the fat, and eliminated it. And that was the beginning of creating my defatted haven . . . Okay, now tell me what you *do* see."

Karen laughed, realizing where Fowler was going. "Okay. Let's see. There's lowfat cream cheese and lowfat mayonnaise, and lowfat Swiss cheese and lowfat mozzarella, and one-percent milk . . . ." She looked up at him. "And I'm beginning to see what you mean."

"Of course you see what I mean. The only full fats I allow in this lowfat haven are some of the *good* fats for adding back, like very good olive oil and canola oil. And even those are in spray containers so I can control how much comes out."

He closed the refrigerator and opened a cupboard door. "And," he said, motioning to the first shelf, "here are all my nuts and seeds. Sunflower, pumpkin, walnuts, pecans, peanuts, and my favorite, almonds, all to have as snacks or to sprinkle on top of my oatmeal and salads and all my amazing stir-fries. And," he said, pointing at a few avocados on the counter, "the occasional avocado, because Janice loves my guacamole."

"I love guacamole too!" Karen exclaimed.

Fowler smiled. "So you see, for me, that's it. That's what I want here, in my haven. This, for now, is the degree to which I want the first habit tailored to my home and my life. The degree I brought it to after deciding, food item by food item, what would work for Janice and me. Because the Power of One Good Habit is not a diet."

Karen, nodding in wonder, said, "It's everything you like to eat. You really do have it your way. When I go on a diet my whole life gets turned around. Nothing I eat is *my* choice. Only the choice of whoever made up the diet. It seems as though my whole life has to accommodate their needs."

Fowler grinned. "That's exactly it. I don't have to accommodate the Power of One Good Habit—it has to accommodate *me*. Here, in my home, each habit accommodates me. And outside of here, in that other world, my habits still accommodate me, because there I adjust them to fit those changed circumstances. That way I can even deal with circumstances that are out of my control."

"So even though a circumstance may be out of your hands," Karen said, repeating the gist of what he had just said, "the Power of One Good Habit never is. You always have control, in every situation, because you control the habits. Right?"

"Exactly! I understand the concept behind each of the eight habits, and that allows me to control them, tailor them to my needs . . . It becomes clearer when you keep reminding yourself of the basics. And what are the basics?"

"That the Power of One Good Habit is not a diet," Karen said quickly.

"Right. That's key. It's not a diet. It's not designed to reach a specific number, then come to an end. What else?"

"That every element of it is flexible?"

Fowler nodded. "That gives it adaptability. The quality to fit your life, at every moment of your life. And next?" he continued. "The big one? The big picture?"

Karen thought for a moment, then shook her head.

Fowler said, "This one I'm going to keep telling you until you see it in your dreams, because this is what we want out of the eight habits every day. Every single day."

"Then wait a second," Karen said. She went back to the table, got her notebook and pen, and returned. "Okay, say it slowly, so I can write it down."

Fowler said, "The goal of the eight habits is to gain health through nutrition—always that—incrementally and continuously, for the rest of our lives. And every step, every tiny step toward that goal, is a success in itself."

Karen wrote it down, carefully, then said, "That is all you want, isn't it? For me to just move in the right direction. Using those small steps. Those easy steps. Steps that can be continually adjusted to fit my life no matter what the situation is."

Fowler nodded, smiling, and Karen went on, "It is a journey, isn't it?" Her thoughts ran ahead of her words. *An almost-pleasant stroll. One step, then another. One success, then another. Use a piece of this habit, a piece of that. Smell the flowers. Take a step. Smile at the neighbors. Take a step. No great sacrifice. No numbers to meet. Nothing to count. Just the step. That's the goal! Take a step, meet your goal. Hello, goal!*

She laughed and said, "And I've already begun! And it was so simple I didn't even realize it! There was no waiting for the right day, no counting down the minutes until I have to go on it. No stuffing my face with all the usual junk, knowing I wouldn't be able to have that great-tasting garbage again until this diet also fails." She smiled. "Those five meals I ate were delicious, and they were the first small steps in the right direction, the first successes. I'm already headed toward nutritional health and losing weight!"

Fowler was watching her, enjoying her sudden burst of insight. Karen laughed again. "Take a step. Then another. For the rest of my life. That's all there is to it. And the first step will lead to the next. And that'll lead to another. And it'll all lead to excitement—the excitement I'm feeling now! And it's that excitement that'll push me forward!"

But even as Fowler was nodding in agreement with her, Karen thought, *Who am I trying to kid? I feel great now, but I know it won't last. This might have worked for you, Fowler, but it's not going to work for me.* She caught herself and shook her head. With a sigh, she said, "I'm sorry, Fowler. I can't . . . I mean, no matter what you say, I still don't think I'll, you know, succeed." She shrugged and again whispered, "Sorry." She waited for Fowler to express his disappointment in her.

Instead, Fowler, suddenly animated, exclaimed, "Perfect! That's perfect! That's the definition of healthy skepticism I was waiting for! Now you're beginning to remind me of myself!"

Karen frowned. She had expected a lecture. "But—"

"No buts, we're rolling here, and it's time for me to tell you about creativity."

"Creativity? Is that one of the habits?"

"No. But it's just as important. Let me put it to you this way—what I'm seeing is our platoon."

"Platoon? We're back to the war?"

"Always! Never forget that." He pulled himself up and backward so he was sitting on the counter. "This is a constant battle, no matter how invisible it becomes. We're fighting those forces out there for our health and the health of the people we love! And our platoon is armed with eight habits, and those habits are so strong, so powerful, that we know with just them we can take on the enemy. But we have even more than the eight habits to rely on. We have two more layers of protection surrounding us, and those layers are defensive, not offensive. One of them is the courage that you already know about, that tiny amount of necessary courage. And the other, within our defensive ring of courage, is creativity. Are you following so far?"

"Yes. And I like it," Karen said, consciously deciding to ignore her doubts and just follow wherever Fowler led. "I'm going to be armed with eight core habits and protected even more by a ring of courage and, within that ring, an inner ring of creativity." Her enthusiasm was coming back. "I know about courage. I know that I don't need much of it, just the tiny amount I'm using now to learn what there is to learn, to take that first tiny step. But what do you mean by creativity?"

"Creativity is just that—being creative. And we've already talked about it. We just didn't define it. But creativity is so important to the Power of One Good Habit that it's got to be defined."

"When did we talk about it?"

"We talked about it when we talked about ways of getting rid of fat. Eliminating egg yolks is creative. Putting our oil into pump sprayers is creative."

"And," Karen said, "eating the meals you gave me to take home, three times in one day, is really creative."

"That's right. Because for us, creativity, when you get right down to it, is the way in which we tailor each of the habits to suit ourselves."

"So what you're saying, then," Karen said, "is that creativity is the quality that gives each of the habits its flexibility. It's how we make each habit our own."

"That's it! The only hard rule with the Power of One Good Habit is that there are *no* hard rules. Each habit, tucked inside a small amount of courage, can be shaped and molded by creativity to fit your needs at every moment."

"But what if I haven't got a creative bone in my body? Which I don't."

"Then you'll still use creativity! But you'll just call it by another name, like wiggle room, or how about this instead of that, or let me test this habit one degree at a time. And then there's my old favorite, that's good enough for today, because it was better than yesterday."

They shared a smile, then Fowler said, "The point I want to make is that creativity, by whatever name, comes into play with every habit."

"Courage to get the war started," Karen said, "Creativity to keep it personally tailored and infinitely mobile. And the habits themselves to wallop the enemy."

"You got it!"

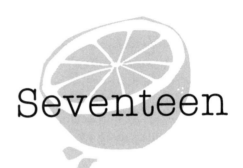

# Seventeen

Courage padded into the room, walked around the counter to Fowler and nudged his hand.

Fowler smiled. "Nature's calling," he said. He began walking toward the door. Then he turned to Karen. "Why don't we go out and take a walk with him in the garden?"

"I'd love to walk through the garden! All I've seen of it so far is the view from the window. Let me just go see how Gabe's doing."

Fowler was on the porch, standing at the railing overlooking the garden, when Karen stepped outside. He was peeling an orange.

Stepping next to him, Karen said, "It's stunning!"

The view from the porch began with a great expanse of manicured lawn that gently sloped to a quarter acre pond filled with hundreds of water lilies. On either side of the lawn and behind the pond, grew a screen of trees, some soaring over fifty feet, others squat and full, creating an impenetrable backdrop. Protected beneath the trees were a collection of multi-hued bushes and flowering shrubs. Woven through all were innumerable varieties of flowers, creating startling splashes of color.

"It looks like a painting," Karen said. "With every tree and bush and flower perfectly placed."

"It's been a thirty-year labor of love," Fowler said, handing half the peeled orange to Karen. "The farm itself is close to thirty acres, most of it fields, none of it in cultivation. But the garden, well, it's closing in on four acres now, and that's about as much as any one person can handle."

"It must be a huge job," Karen said, pulling off an orange section and putting it in her mouth.

Fowler nodded. "From March to October it doesn't let you take much time off, that's true; but the way it's designed, a lot of it really takes care of itself." He motioned Karen down the stairs and to a cobblestone walk that curved toward a spectacular weeping willow. "Take these borders, for example. They're designed so I can easily cut them with just one pass of my riding mower. Made so I can get right up to the perennial beds without even slowing down. There's no fussiness about it, not like some of your city gardens."

Karen was taking in the spectacular view.

"I like to look at the garden the same way I look at the eight habits," Fowler continued. "You know, it's got to fit in. Fit me. No part of it can take more of my time than I think it's worth. Otherwise it begins to gnaw at my nerves." He finished his half of the orange.

"I never realized that making something disappear into your life could take so much forethought." Karen said. She too ate the last piece of orange.

"Now you're talking about the Power of One Good Habit, aren't you?"

Karen laughed. "Lately, that's all I think about—the Power of One Good Habit, and food. But not in the way you do."

"Oh yeah? Tell me about that," Fowler said, turning to her. "Tell me how you start your food day."

"You mean breakfast?"

Fowler nodded. "Breakfast on a workday."

Again Karen laughed. "There *is* no breakfast on a workday! It's impossible. First there's Gary. Getting him out of the house. Taking care of whatever he needs. And Gabe: getting him ready for the sitter, then dropping him off at her house, then driving into town and hopefully getting to the office by nine."

"So what time is it when you do have your first meal in the morning?" Fowler asked.

Karen shrugged. "I'd say about ten, ten-fifteen. That's when I get a doughnut and coffee from the snack bar in the building."

Courage ran across an open section of lawn. Fowler laughed and pointed. "He likes to lord it over the squirrels, tell 'em who's boss." Then facing Karen again, he said, "We talked about creativity, so now I want you to work with me. To find your creative streak."

Karen nodded. "Okay."

"If you wanted," Fowler continued, "could you have your doughnut and coffee earlier?"

Without hesitation Karen replied, "Sure. I could have it as soon as I walk into the office. Just pick it up on the way in and eat it at my desk, like everyone else. Except that early in the morning, I'm not really hungry. And let's face it, the less I eat, the better. So I don't. I just wait—and hope that one day all that waiting will add up to the loss of a pound or two."

Fowler said, "I'll let you in on a little secret. Skipping breakfast contributes to weight gain, while eating breakfast contributes to weight loss." He smiled at the puzzled expression on Karen's face and said, "The second habit is: You have to include breakfast every day."

"But why?" Karen said. "I don't understand. How can *not*

eating cause me to gain weight, and eating cause me to lose weight? It doesn't make sense."

"It's like this," Fowler said, directing Karen onto another path, this one heading to the back of the pond. "A large part of the work our body does in a twenty-four-hour period is digest our food, break down the carbs and proteins and fats we eat into the nutrients our body needs. And it does most of this work during the day, while we're awake. In fact, it does it *best* while we're awake. And while our body is digesting this food, while it's *working* at that, it's burning calories. And when it burns calories, we lose weight. Because that's what weight loss is—the burning of enough calories."

"So you're saying that I need to eat breakfast to get my body to start working? To start digesting food?"

"Exactly. The most efficient time for our body to digest food is during the day. And it begins this work as soon as we eat breakfast: the first meal of the day. Because without breakfast, there's nothing for it to digest. So if we eat breakfast first thing in the morning, our body begins working first thing in the morning, and begins burning calories first thing in the morning, and that makes it begin losing weight first thing in the morning." Fowler smiled. "Maybe I can explain it to you this way. Remember when I said the food we eat is our fuel, same as the fuel in our cars?"

"Sure."

"So, starting first thing in the morning, and for the rest of the day, think of it as though we're using our car. Our body is our car. And because we're using it, we need to put in fuel. In fact, we need to constantly make sure it has enough fuel to keep running. And we do this until the end of the day, when we let the fuel tank close in on empty, because we know we're about to park the car for the night, and this type of car just doesn't like to have its tank full while it's parked. While we sleep."

He bent, picked up a pebble, and tossed it into the pond. "The next morning, though, when we wake up, the car—our body, without fuel—is basically shut down. Oh sure, the light for the alarm still blinks and the clock still works. You can breathe and talk and take care of Gabe. But the essentials on the inside are at a standstill. The car is parked. It's sitting in the garage. And none of the really important work gets done because you're not burning enough calories. And without that, you're not losing weight. Here's the thing though: you *can't* burn those calories until you give the car more fuel to burn. That's why you have to feed it breakfast. Breakfast is the key that lets you crank your car's ignition and press down hard on the gas. It starts your engine. Gets everything going again."

Courage came running up to them. Fowler said to the dog, "Go on! Do your thing!" And snapped his fingers. The dog ran off, disappearing into the trees.

Fowler smiled at Karen.

Karen, though, her brow creased in thought, said, "But what if I'm not hungry first thing in the morning? Which is the case most days. What do I do then? How can I eat breakfast if I'm not hungry?"

"The answer to that starts the night before," Fowler said. "Tell me, when is the last time you eat in the evening?"

Karen thought for a moment before saying, "The last time I eat is usually late. Right before bedtime. Sometimes I'll even have my last snack in bed."

"Well there's your answer. That's why you're not hungry at breakfast. The key to feeling hungry in the morning, to needing breakfast, is to stop eating at a certain time in the evening. That way your body can finish digesting all you've eaten long before you get up. Think of it this way: you want to park the car with the fuel indicator on empty. That way you wake up hungry, needing fuel, needing to eat breakfast. In fact, I just read a study that showed how people who eat breakfast regularly eat on average one hundred fewer calories a day. And that's because eating breakfast makes them less likely to overeat at lunch or dinner, or even at their evening snack. And though a one-hundred-calorie savings doesn't sound like much, in a year it adds up to the loss of ten pounds."

"Ten pounds!"

"You bet. Ten hip-hugging, chin-hanging pounds."

"Okay," Karen said, beginning to sound as though she was getting it. "Let's see if I have it right. I have to eat breakfast, it's an important meal. And the key to eating breakfast, the key to getting my body to start burning calories and start losing weight first thing in the morning, which is when it begins to burn calories best, is to stop eating at a certain time before I go to bed."

"You got it," Fowler said. "Look, before I started applying this habit, I also used to eat right up to bedtime. Then I'd have trouble falling asleep because I'd feel full and uncomfortable. You know, like a sack of potatoes was stuffed into my stomach. So of course in the morning I'd wake up not hungry. Then I'd step on the scale and see that I'd gained weight. But now, because I stop eating a few hours before I go to bed, it's just the opposite. And there's nothing special about when I stop. There's no rules. No watching the clock or anything like that. I just keep the thought in the back of my head that I don't want to go to sleep feeling full."

"But what if I'm hungry before bedtime? Do I have to go to sleep hungry?"

"Not at all. In fact, if you're anything like me, you can't fall asleep if you're hungry. What I do in that case is have a very light snack; a piece of fruit or a small bowl of cereal or just a slice of lowfat cheese. Even just a few almonds can do the trick. All I need is something light to take the edge off my hunger so I can sleep. To tell you the truth, most nights a glass of water with lemon or a cup of herbal tea does the trick." He motioned to another bend in the path, saying, "This'll take us past the rose garden, and then back to the house."

"It really is beautiful," Karen said. "I feel as though I'm in a different country. Someplace exotic!" She laughed, then in a serious tone, added, "You know, this is the first time I've really understood how the calorie-burning process *begins*. Really, how losing weight begins." She started ticking off points on her fingers. "The body has to digest its food. And when it does, it's working. So we lose weight. And because it digests its food best during the day, beginning first thing in the morning, I have to stop eating at a certain time at night, so I can wake up feeling hungry. Because if I feel hungry I'm going to want to eat breakfast. And breakfast, again, is what gets my body to start the day off right, by losing weight . . . When you think about it, it's a perfect circle. Everything works toward the same goal of losing weight. And none of it's about starving. In fact, it's the opposite. It's all about eating!"

Fowler turned to Karen. "That has got to be the best description of the weight-loss process I've ever heard or read! And that's also the second habit. And if you use just the two habits you now know, to the degree they fit your circumstances, you'll lose weight. Without a doubt, you'll lose weight. But losing weight isn't the point."

"No," Karen agreed, remembering Fowler's mantra. "Losing weight isn't the point. The point is gaining health. But," she added, "losing weight would be so, so . . . "

"Exciting?"

"You'd better believe it!"

"I do believe it. In fact, I still feel it every day, every morning when I look in the mirror, every morning when I walk into the restaurant and see those trousers on the wall."

Karen's eyes were shining. "Okay, then. My second habit: include breakfast every day. And stop eating two or three hours before going to bed so I'll be hungry in the morning. And now, with my new creative streak, I can start my day by picking up breakfast on the way in to the office and eat it at nine o'clock."

"Eat what?" Fowler asked.

"Eat my . . . " She paused, thought for a moment, then said, laughing, "Eat my fried-in-lard, filled-with-fat doughnut. Or else I could order a bagel, or toast, spread with lowfat cream cheese."

"That's it!" Fowler replied. "Just make the bagel or bread whole wheat or whole grain."

"Or," Karen said, her mind racing, "I can have an orange like today or a banana with lowfat yogurt or a piece of lowfat cheese, or even one of your delicious meals meant for supper."

"Now that's more like it!" Fowler said. "And when you include that lowfat yogurt or cheese, or any other lowfat protein, it not only helps keep your blood sugar steady all morning, but also helps manage your mid-morning hunger pangs. It even goes a long way toward stopping those irritating energy and mood swings we can get."

"What! Just having some protein for breakfast can do all that? Work on my energy and mood swings?"

"It sure can," Fowler said. "Janice and I have diabetes in the family, so knowing this is important to us. And really, it's important to everyone. That's why I have this protein message branded on my brain."

With a touch to her shoulder Fowler indicated that Karen should slow down. He said, "When we get past this wall of shrubbery, look to your right."

"Oh, my!" Karen said, stepping beyond the shrubs. "This is . . . just . . . amazing!"

"My rose garden," Fowler said. For a moment he let Karen take in the magnificent view, then he walked a few feet into a narrow path between the rose bushes and cupped one rose in particular in his palm. He motioned Karen to come closer. "This one's very unusual. In fact, it's one-of-a-kind, because I hybridized it myself."

"Gorgeous! Just beautiful!" Karen said, gently touching the large pink, red and yellow bloom. She bent over to take in its scent.

"I call it the Precious Janice," Fowler said. His eyes began to moisten.

Karen put her hand on Fowler's arm. "She's a wonderful woman. Just wonderful And she's so lucky to have you."

"No," Fowler said, "It's the other way around. I'm the lucky one."

They gazed at the rose garden for another minute or two, then Fowler said, "We should get going . . . " And he motioned Karen back on to the path. Putting two fingers to his mouth he whistled sharply. A moment later Courage was at his side. "Home!" he said. In a flash the dog was gone.

They walked a few steps in silence, then Karen said, "Why doesn't everyone know all that you're telling me about eating? About how everything works? This information is so important these days. And so basic. We should be learning it the way we learn that smoking is bad for us." Then she added, "You know, when you think about it, what we're talking about is really so simple. Stop eating in the evening, at no special time, just two or three hours before bed. Then, the next morning, eat breakfast. Just that. And remember about the fat and the protein. No big deal. Just keep the thought of stopping in my mind at night, and of putting something quick and easy into my mouth in the morning. And for that the lowfat choices are there, the protein choices. And they're so easily available. No big deal. Nothing to obsess about. Practically nothing to even think about."

"That's something else I was waiting to hear from you," Fowler said. "It's what dawned on me a long time ago. It's not a big deal. None of it. Nothing to obsess over. Because with the Power of One Good Habit, there is nothing to get obsessed about."

"You're right," Karen said. "But you want to know something? At this moment I am looking forward to losing weight by eating a healthy breakfast every morning. And to not going to bed on a full stomach every night. Because this time I know I can do it. I really can!"

They crested a small hill, then stepped through a funnel of box hedge. From here they could see a corner of the house.

"Every bend of this path exposes another world," Karen said. "And everything looks as though it's been here for a thousand years."

Fowler smiled. "I like to have the garden blend into the landscape, until the landscape begins to flow from the garden. They become one—the garden, the distant trees, the sky. You know, no lines, no breaks."

"That sounds like the Power of One Good Habit," Karen said.

Fowler grinned. "The similarity is not accidental."

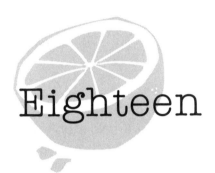

# Eighteen

"Okay," Fowler said to Karen once they were back on the lawn and headed to the house. "We talked about breakfast at work, so now tell me what your usual breakfast at home looks like."

They could see Courage sitting on the back porch, waiting for them.

Karen, shrugging, said, "My usual breakfast? That's simple enough. If I have anything more than coffee, it'll be a bowl of Sweet Smacks or a toaster pastry or two." She turned to Fowler and laughed at the sudden, exaggerated look of shock on his face. "What? What happened? What did I say?"

"What you said," Fowler answered, "was the cue for me to give you the next habit: Tame your sweet tooth!"

For a moment Karen only looked at Fowler. Then she said, shaking her head, "Tame my sweet tooth? Well, here it is. Here, for me, is where the Power of One Good Habit falls apart."

"It won't."

"It will! You just don't *know*. My sweet tooth is the size of New York!"

"And mine used to be the size of Texas," Fowler said calmly. "Until I tamed it. Until I taught myself how to cut down my need for sugar."

"You can do that? How? How does that work?"

"I'll tell you how. But first I want to tell you *why*. Even though sugar is a carb, it's an empty carb, a carb filled with useless calories. No—not just useless calories, *dangerous* calories. And if we go back to my old clunker . . . "

"Where carbs are the fuel," Karen said.

"Right. Where carbs are the fuel. *Sugar* carbs are the exception. Putting sugar into our body would be like adding jet fuel to my car! It's way too concentrated. Sugar forces our body to make insulin, which shoves all that sugar into our cells. And that can cause a sugar overload."

"A what?"

"A sugar overload. A two-barreled shotgun blast that'll make you gain weight with the first cartridge, and lead to insulin resistance and type-two diabetes with the second. Just like that. Pow! Pow! And diabetes is a killer. I know that from my own family."

"My family, too," Karen said.

"There you go," Fowler continued, "And just like fat, sugar is also a master of disguise, coming in all shapes and colors and sizes. Always trying to find its way into your life."

"And onto my second chin," Karen added with a smile.

"Sounds like you've met sugar before."

"Have I ever!" Karen said. "He's the sweetest guy in my life." She laughed at herself for a moment, then turned her head so Fowler wouldn't be able to read her expression, see what was in her eyes. *Please, Gary*, she thought. *We can get through this.* She turned back to Fowler, forcing a smile. "Okay. Tell me more about sugar."

Courage began to bark. Fowler laughed, saying, "If he's away from Janice for a few minutes longer than usual, he goes nuts. Okay, sugar, well, if there's anything good to say about sugar, it's that it's easier to find than fat. Because the test for sugar is that it's sweet."

"My toaster pastries," Karen said, shaking her head. "And my doughnut at work. And the Sweet Smacks in the morning."

"Exactly. Toaster pastries and Sweet Smacks and especially all those sugar-filled drinks like sodas. So, since this habit is geared to real life and based on common sense, the test for sugar is, if something's sweet and it's not a fruit, then it's filled with sugar.

"What about sugar substitutes? Those are sweet. And they're not sugar."

Fowler smiled. "I spent a lot of time thinking about sugar substitutes. To tell you the truth, Janice and I talked that subject to death. And the answer we came up with was, sure, in some cases sugar substitutes work, because of course they're better than high-calorie sugar. But relying on sugar substitutes is really missing the point of this habit, because this habit says to *tame* your sweet tooth, not to fool it. And using sugar substitutes doesn't do anything to dial down the level of sweetness your taste buds are programmed for."

"Can you really do that?" Karen asked. "Tame your sweet tooth? There are times when my urge for something sweet just drives me mad!"

"You and me both," Fowler said. "And that's why this habit was designed to work on that. On taming your sweet tooth, not just on telling you to *avoid* sweets. There's a big difference between the two. This habit will get your taste buds to say they don't want that high level of sweetness any more. Get you to not like that much sweetness. It'll work the same way that lowering the fat content will get you to not like so much fat. And that's its true strength. Once you don't want that sugary taste any more, you won't feel deprived. So you'll just naturally start eating less sugar. It'll be as though an invisible force is now operating inside you, pushing away that urge for sweets. With this habit, before you know it, your sweet tooth *will* be tamed."

"Okay," Karen said, sounding skeptical. "So how does it work? What kind of fiery hoops do I have to jump through?"

Fowler smiled. They walked up the stairs to the back porch and he opened the door for Karen, allowing Courage to dash in first. "No hoops," he said. "Fiery or otherwise. All you have to do is like eating something fresh, delicious and sweet. And to make sure I don't forget to do that, I keep it as the centerpiece on both my coffee and kitchen table."

Karen, stepping into the kitchen, said, "The fruit bowl?"

"You bet! Nature's own cure for a sweet tooth. Tell me, do you like fruit?"

"Yes. Sure. So does Gary."

"Good. And how many fruits a day do you eat?"

"A day? One . . . maybe. If it's there. I never really think about fruit."

Fowler grinned. "You sound like me, a hundred pounds ago. Then, because of Janice, I started using fruit to my advantage." He picked up an apple, a pear and a peach. "The magic number for fruit is three. Three a day. Just for you. And it doesn't matter if it's for dessert or a snack or for breakfast. And remember: don't hide them in the fridge. Keep them in sight and within reach, even at work. That'll take care of your sweet tooth. Three a day, that's twenty-one in a week. Just for you. And another twenty-one for Gary. So you're on a major hunt for fruit when you go shopping. Work on it for seven days, and *then* talk to me about your sweet tooth!"

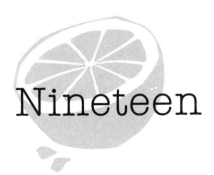

# Nineteen

"Now," Fowler said, "It's time for me to take you on another tour of my restaurant."

"Just give me a minute," Karen said, "so I can go see if Gabe's up."

Janice was just closing down her computer. "Perfect timing," she said. "For Gabe too. He opened his eyes a few minutes ago. I think he was going to cry, but as soon as I started talking to him he seemed to forget about that. Maybe it's my voice. He's never heard one like mine before."

Karen picked up the baby. Gabe put his arms around her neck, but his eyes were on Janice. "Maybe it is your voice," she said. "But by now it's not that he finds it unusual, it's that he finds it comforting. Not just your voice, but you."

"You think so?" Janice said, excitedly, pressing the lever on her wheelchair and steering it to the door.

"Of course! Just look at him. I think he's in love."

"Finished?" Fowler asked Janice as she came into the

kitchen. She was wearing a wide smile. Courage was at her side. Karen and Gabe were right behind her.

"What?" Fowler said to her. "Why are you smiling?"

"Because I have a boyfriend," Janice said. She laughed. So did Karen.

Karen said, "It's Gabe. He can't take his eyes off Janice."

Fowler smiled, then said to Janice, "How did it go? Are you getting anywhere?

Janice shook her head. "Some people just don't want to listen to reason." She turned to Karen. "For the past hour I was online with five people from four countries in two time zones. All of us are worried about the rush to genetically modified foods. If I had my way, there'd be very little of it commercially available, at least until the studies are more conclusive."

"It's already much more widespread than most people realize," Fowler said, adding, "I just told Karen how to cure her sweet tooth."

"Good!" Janice said, turning to Karen. "Before he figured this trick out, his cravings were so strong that if there was nothing sweet in the house, I would catch him in the kitchen swigging corn syrup."

"That's incredible!" Karen said, even though she knew her own urges were just as strong as Fowler's.

Gabe let out a tentative cry. Karen, rocking him slightly, said, "Uh-oh. I think someone needs changing."

"May I help?" Janice asked.

"Of course."

Karen carried Gabe to the spare bedroom and placed him on the bed. While Janice played with his hands, Karen changed his diaper. "See," she said. "Look how relaxed he is with you. That's unusual for him. He's already at the point where he's becoming wary of strangers."

"But he's a quiet baby, isn't he? I mean, he's not very fussy."

"Only when he's showing off, like now," Karen said, laughing. "At home he can be a little devil. She smiled at the expression of delight on Janice's face as Gabe reached for her fingers.

When they returned to the kitchen, they found Fowler whistling along to a tune on the radio. "Okay," Karen said, placing Gabe, now practicing his bubble-blowing, into his seat. "I'm ready for that tour of your restaurant. Just give me a couple of minutes to see if Gabe's hungry." She buckled in the baby, saying, "Did you tell Janice that you're now sitting in a high chair at home?"

"Is that a new development?" Janice asked, guiding her chair next to Gabe.

"It is, and it's great for me. Makes it a lot easier at meal-time." Karen reached for her baby tote bag and took out a jar of food and a small plastic spoon.

"What's that?" Janice asked.

"Sweet potato. It's new for him." She opened the jar, dipped in the spoon, and brought it to the baby's lips. He opened his mouth and she put a small amount on his tongue. He swallowed it, then squealed loudly, his arms flapping.

"He likes it!" Karen said, then turning to Janice, she asked, "Would you like to feed him? I'm supposed to go on another tour of your father's restaurant."

"Oh yes! I'd be happy to."

"Good. Just put small amounts on his tongue, and let him eat until he doesn't want any more."

She watched as Janice fed Gabe a couple of spoonfuls of the sweet potato, then stepped into the cooking area, saying to Fowler, "It looks like he's in very capable hands. Okay, tour time. What do you want me to do?"

"What I want you to do first," Fowler said playfully, "is to think of finding sugar . . . in terms of a party!" He laughed.

"A party? I thought we were fighting a war?"

"We *are* fighting a war! But at the moment we're not just ordinary soldiers, we're highly trained spies. We're James Bond!"

Janice laughed.

Karen raised her brows, her smile too, growing. "James Bond and Jane Bond!"

"Right!" Fowler said. "James and Jane. And we're at this party in . . . "

"Tangier!"

"That's it. Now you're getting it. Can you feel the intrigue? The undercurrent of powerful forces?"

"Good versus evil!" Janice chimed in.

"Exactly," Fowler said, "Good versus evil. And we're the good guys."

"Of course," Karen said.

"And the bad guys are . . . ?" Fowler asked.

"Sugar!"

"Right! But they're devious, those bad sugars, because they're trying to . . . "

"Seduce us!" Karen said.

"That's it!" Fowler answered. "They want to seduce us. But they can't unless we let them, because we know who they are. They're the noisiest, brashest, most exciting people at the party. They're uninhibited, dance to the most intense beats, laugh the loudest."

"They're the most fun to be with!"

"That they are," Fowler replied. "But . . . ?"

"But? But what?" Karen asked.

"Come on, Jane Bond," Fowler said. "Work with me here."

Karen, fumbling, said, "But we're too smart for them?"

"That's right. We are too smart for them. How are we too smart for them?"

"We're too smart for them because we know what they want."

"Exactly! And what do they want?"

"They want us to take them home so they can get under our skin and live on our hips."

"Right!" Fowler said. "But we won't let that happen, because now that we know who they are, we're going to do our job, do what we're trained for: we're going to take them out!"

125

"Search and destroy!"

"That's it! And we'll begin by leaving those bad sugars at the party and taking home only the good guys," Fowler said, opening a cupboard door.

"Hey!" Karen said. "A jar of sugar! You just said we have to leave sugar at the party in Tangier."

Janice laughed. She said to Gabe, "Your mom and my dad are cuckoo!"

Fowler said, "Karen, remember what I told you. The habits are designed to be tailored to each of us, to fit our individual needs, because we're not all stamped from the same mold. So even though the habits give all of us identical guidelines, the way we each apply those guidelines will vary. And in my case, though the habit says to have as little sugar as possible, I personally enjoy a cup of tea in the afternoon."

"So very British."

"Yes. It is. And I also refuse to have my tea without sugar."

For a moment Karen looked puzzled. Then she suddenly realized that what Fowler had just said was almost unbelievable. She looked directly at him and said, "You know, you said that so quickly, and gave it so little importance. But just think what it means. You said you *allow* yourself sugar in your tea. That it's *your choice*. That this is the way *you* tailored this habit to fit *your* needs."

"Exactly," Fowler said. "I'm still following what the habit says, but I do it on my own terms. I refuse to struggle with it, and so I don't."

Karen shook her head in amazement. "You know, at every turn it hits me over and over that the Power of One Good Habit isn't a diet. That it really doesn't have that all-or-nothing diet mentality. It is a guideline, isn't it? One that everyone's been missing. It's a true return to nutritional sanity."

"I couldn't have put it better myself," Fowler said. "But another thing you should know about that teaspoon of sugar in my tea is that it used to be four teaspoons, even five."

"Wow."

"Yes. Then I started to get smart, started to apply what I was learning, and I began to dial down how much I was using, to begin getting that need for so much sugar out of my system."

"He was worried about diabetes," Janice said.

"I was, and we all should be, for ourselves and our kids. So I used my fruit and my fear of diabetes to begin a slow but steady decrease of how much sugar I used, until I got it *exactly* where I wanted. In fact, if I were to put four teaspoons of sugar in my tea today, I wouldn't be able to drink it! I've lost my taste for that much sweetening."

"The way you lost your taste for fat?" Karen asked.

"Exactly. You can lose your taste for sugar the same way you can lose your taste for fat. The key is to just dial it down, one notch at a time. One teaspoon at a time. One type of sugary food at a time." Then he said, waving his arm impatiently, "All right! Enough about sugar, let's continue with that tour!" He opened the rest of the cupboard doors, saying, "Okay, tell me what else you see, and when we've finished that, I'll tell you about the fourth habit."

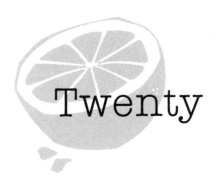

# Twenty

"Yes!" Karen said to Fowler. "The fourth habit." Then she said, "Okay. First you want me to tell you what else I see. Well, I see one bottle of olive oil, and another of canola, and the two pump sprayers you put them into. And that little jar of sugar . . . "

"Right. And?"

"And . . . that's about it. That's all I see that applies to the first three habits—finding the fat, taming my sweet tooth and including breakfast every day. Of course I also see whole multi-grain bread and multi-grain rolls. Cans of chickpeas and beans and lentils. Tuna and salmon and tomatoes. All different types of whole-grain pastas and brown rice and wild rice . . . "

Turning to the refrigerator and deli counter she continued, "And there's plenty of vegetables and precut veggies with dip. And salad and one-percent milk and all those low-fat cheeses and yogurt. And both raw eggs and hard-boiled eggs, and, of course, that huge bowl of fruit on the table. Whew!"

Fowler was smiling. "You're not done yet. What about the freezer?"

Karen opened the door. "Okay. Here I see all sorts of frozen vegetables. Packages of turkey breasts, ground turkey, and chicken breasts." She moved a package over a little. "And there's veal and ground meat and all your banked meals . . . "

"Okay," Fowler said, "now that you saw what *is* there, I want you to tell me what *isn't* there."

Karen looked at Janice. "He is strange, isn't he?"

Janice though, was focused on Gabe. Karen could see she had finished feeding him, and without needing to ask directions, had taken out a wet towelette from Karen's bag and wiped Gabe's face and hands. Now she was smiling and listening to one of his babbled stories while he held her thumb in his hand. Karen said, more loudly, "Janice, your father wants to know what I don't see in his restaurant."

"What you don't see," Janice said to Karen, "is any processed or chemically enhanced meals or snacks."

"What?" Karen turned back to look at the freezer's contents.

"That's right," Fowler said. "Remember when I told you there are three very different groups involved in producing the food we eat? And I said the first group is responsible for growing and harvesting all our natural food, the kind of food I like to think of as being close to the farm?"

"I remember that," Karen said, nodding. She closed the freezer door and leaned against the counter. "And you said the second group is the one that takes that natural food and turns it into products that are nutritious, that don't compromise our health."

"That's right," Fowler said. "And then there's the third group, the one that, unfortunately, takes that natural food and processes it into products that contain excess fat and sugar and added chemicals."

He shrugged. "So what you *won't* see in my restaurant,

my haven, are those processed foods. Processed meals and snacks." He paused, then repeated with even more emphasis, "Here, in my restaurant, there are no chemically enhanced foods with ingredients my body doesn't need, with ingredients I can't pronounce or items whose source I can't figure out. Here, everything we have, within reason, is as close to natural, or as close to the farm, as possible. And that's not to say I don't want anything that comes in cans or boxes or bags or jars. It's not the *containers* I object to, it's what's in them! In my haven, as much as possible, I want the primary source of food, and not the food that that third group processes it into."

Karen said, "No processed meals or snacks." She thought about this for a moment, wincing. "Let me tell you, in my kitchen, I have them all! Frozen meals, meals in boxes, pouches of prepared pastas and rice. Oh, and chips and cookies and doughnuts and everything else under the sun that's greasy and sugar-filled."

Then her eyes widened as she realized what Fowler had been getting at all along. "It really is all the same, isn't it? The processed food in my kitchen is the same as the food I get at the fast-food joints or family restaurants, or when I order in. Same junk, different names. They're the enemy's weapons, advertised to the hilt and aimed right at my house. Right at my family!"

"That's exactly what they are," Fowler said. "But we forget that, because if we have to put it into a pot or heat it up in the microwave, it feels different. It feels as though we're making it ourselves."

Janice said," After a speech like that, can you tell what the fourth habit is?"

"Boy, can I ever! Habit Number Four: Replace processed or chemically enhanced foods with wholesome close-to-the-farm foods." Then Karen added, "Within reason."

"According to your carefully thought-out needs, tastes, and circumstances," Fowler said.

"According to my needs, tastes, and circumstances,"

Karen repeated, knowing that up to now her needs said she had to have her kitchen filled with white sandwich breads and prepared meals and snacks—the eat-right-out-of-the-bag kind, the heat-up kind, the open-the-can-or-pouch-and-throw-it-into-a-pot-and-hope-for-the-best kind. All necessary for those times when she was rushed or tired or just not in the mood to cook.

Then she had a thought. *Why is that? Why can't I also replace that junk with nutritious meals and snacks of my own, the way Fowler does? Fill up my cupboards with the ingredients for meals that can be made in minutes, the way his cupboards are filled? And save portions of meals in the freezer for other times instead of relying on the processed stuff? What's so wrong with me, that's so right with him?* She shook her head. *Gary says it's that I'm lazy, even stupid. But that's not true. It's just that I didn't have the answer. Until this minute, I didn't realize there was another way.*

To Fowler she said, "It really is a war, isn't it? I'm fighting the enemy, and at the same time I'm also fighting against myself! But I can defeat them and change *me*. I know it! Change the way I shop, change the way I cook. I can use all the concepts of the eight habits and fit them into my life the way you did, make them fit my needs and circumstances!"

She smiled. "There is a certain excitement to all this, isn't there? Whether you call it the beginning of a journey or fighting a war, it does get the adrenaline pumping." Then she thought, *there's even another benefit to this*, and she added, "You know, if you think about it, not buying all those processed snacks and meals means leaving out whole aisles in the grocery store. It might even save money."

"It will," Fowler promised. "But that bonus is completely beside the point. The reason for having this habit is that it gives us control over our own nutritional lives. It gives us control over killers like trans fat. And it gives us control over ingredients like salt. It takes that power away from the enemy and places it back in our hands. This habit makes me feel powerful."

"I think," Janice said to Fowler, "that this habit was the one you thought about most. It's the one you kept honing, kept digging deeper into. The one that, long after you'd accepted its basic tenets, you still found yourself searching through, always trying to discover your bottom-line comfort level."

"You're right," Fowler agreed. "I do it all so unconsciously now, so naturally. But I remember when everything I bought, everything I brought into the restaurant, I analyzed. Thought it through. Decided whether it was up to my ever-increasing standards."

Karen had found her notebook and was taking notes again at the counter. She said, "You first developed the concept of this habit, then looked at it degree by degree, item by item, until you came to the point you're at now, what you call your comfort level?"

"That's it," Fowler said. Then, walking to the refrigerator and opening one of its drawers, he added, "Talking about my comfort level, you haven't looked in here yet."

Karen stepped closer. "What's this?" she asked, lifting out a package of meatless, soy-based pepperoni. "This is certainly a processed food."

"That's what I mean about adjusting to your comfort level," Fowler said. "One of my favorite foods used to be pepperoni pizza, especially if it was dripping with fat. And I didn't want to give it up. So I didn't! I still have it, often. But now I make it—you'd be amazed at how simple it is to make. I cook several at a time and freeze them." He gestured toward the package in Karen's hands. "But, you see, to make them the way I like them, I need this product, this factory-made product, which I think is excellent. So I buy it all the time, along with lowfat mozzarella cheese and canned pizza sauce and mushrooms and green peppers. And I challenge any store-bought or ordered-in pizza to a taste test against mine." He grinned. "But mine, unlike theirs, is downright healthy."

Karen said, "It's amazing how adjustable the habits are. So unlike a diet. They really do let you move forward gradually, at a pace *anyone* can live with, instead of a pace someone else decides. I only know four of the eight habits so far, but even with that, I don't know if I can ever really eat the way I did before. At least not without feeling that something's wrong. When it's so easy to get . . . " She looked at her notes. "When it's so easy to gain health—always that, incrementally and continuously, for the rest of your life." Then she added, "And so easy to lose weight. Especially that!"

"Not especially that," Fowler said. "Though I have to admit, when I first started this for myself, weight loss was the goal. But I can see now that that goal was shortsighted. With my focus only on losing weight, I was denying myself something much more important. And that's health. Mine and Janice's."

He took the package from Karen and put it back into the refrigerator. "But that doesn't mean I don't know what you're feeling. Seeing your blood pressure go down, your blood sugar stabilize, your cholesterol drop, your chances of diabetes and heart disease and cancer lessen—at certain times, all that seems like small potatoes compared to looking in the mirror and beginning to like what you see. For me, when that happened, when I was able to look in the mirror and say, 'There, that's more like it,' it was nothing short of exceptional!"

—

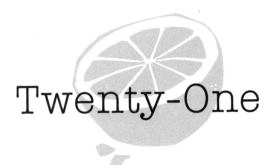

# Twenty-One

"All right," Fowler said, clapping his hands. "Time to eat! To have our lazy, Sunday-morning, Power of One Good Habit fantasy breakfast—on a Monday!"

"Great!" Karen said excitedly. But her expression suddenly changed, and with a puzzled look she added, "I know we just talked about processed and chemically enhanced foods . . . And now we're going to be eating breakfast . . . So, what about cereals? I mean . . . You know, the fat-free and sugar-free brands, served with skim or one-percent milk? Would that be all right?"

"You tell me," Fowler said.

Karen's brow creased. "Well, if they're low in fat and low in sugar . . . "

"And made from whole grains," Fowler added.

"And made from whole grains," Karen repeated.

"And don't have added food colorings and artificial flavorings . . . " Janice said.

Karen's eyes widened. "And don't have added chemical enhancers that love to hide out in the cereal aisle!" She laughed. "Then I'd say yes, they would be all right."

"Not just all right," Fowler said, opening the cupboard next to the refrigerator and pointing at a box of shredded wheat and another of bran flakes and a third of Kashi, "but excellent! Karen, I'll say this again, because it's at the core of what I'm teaching you. The eight habits are based on real life and common sense! And when a product is good, it's good." He reached for one of the cereal boxes and pointed to the nutrition label. "It's all here. On every package. You just have to take a look at what's available. Assess it for its nutritional value, for your lifestyle, for your immediate circumstances, and then make your choice."

"It really is simple!" Karen exclaimed.

Fowler thought a moment before saying, "The eight habits are simple in theory. That's true. And they're simple when they finally become second nature. When the thought of going back to your old way of eating is impossible. But at the beginning . . . No. And that's why, once you take your first step, adopt the first habit, achieve that first success—"

"And then the next and the next!" Karen said.

"That's right, and then the next and the next, and given all eight habits the time they need to build momentum, to become an integral part of your life, you can proudly hold your head up high in victory."

"Victory at having beaten the enemy!"

"Exactly."

Karen was beaming.

"Okay!" Fowler said. "Now let's go all-out. Today we have the time and the company. So you tell me *your* dream breakfast. And Janice will tell us hers. And I'll tell you mine. Because the way each of us applies the habits will be different. It'll be uniquely our own, dictated by our personal tastes. Then together we'll create courageous and creative magic!"

"Okay," Karen said. "My dream breakfast? That's easy. What I feel like eating right now is a western omelet with home-fried potatoes and a ton of bacon."

"Okay," Janice said to Fowler, laughing. "Let's see you get out of that one!"

"Well, the spuds are on. And they'll be perfection. And the omelet too, you can count on that also being outstanding. And the bacon? Later I'll tell you how you can have the bacon and still be within the boundaries of the habits, because within the eight habits, no food is left out. But for today, since bacon doesn't fit into my lowfat haven, the one I designed for *me*, the best I can do is find you a perfectly acceptable replacement."

"You know," Karen said, "knowing I can have everything except the bacon, makes the bacon itself seem insignificant."

"Aha! Now, looking at food from that perspective," Fowler said, "is courage." He turned to his daughter, his eyebrows raised. "You?"

Janice said, "I'll have a cheese omelet."

"Good. And for me, I know exactly what I want. I've been thinking about it all morning—spaghetti and meat sauce with scrambled eggs and turkey balls."

"What!" Karen gasped.

Janice said to her, "He's not kidding. He can have his dinner in the morning and his breakfast at night, or just pizza three times a day. I've never been able to understand his cravings or his appetite."

Fowler smiled at Karen. "To our bodies, food is just a bunch of nutrients. As long as what you're eating follows the concepts of the habits, it doesn't matter what label you think the meal should have—breakfast, lunch, dinner or snack. So let's get to work! We have VIP customers, and we're going to knock their socks off!"

Then, his words rapid, he said, "Why don't you start by refilling our glasses with water and lemon? Then put the kettle on for tea. Then clean a green pepper and a handful of mushrooms, and grab a couple of spuds from the pantry and let's get them peeled."

"Yes, sir!" Karen answered.

Working beside her, Fowler took a carton of eggs and two large packages of regular ground beef from the refrigerator.

"Even *I* know that that meat is filled with fat," Karen said.

"Watch and learn," Fowler countered. He opened the packages of ground beef, dropped them into a large pot, set the pot on the stove with the burner adjusted to medium and began breaking up the meat with a wooden spoon.

Karen, keeping one eye on Fowler, washed the green pepper and mushrooms, diced them, then began to peel the potatoes, saying, "Do you ever use sweet potatoes? I remember reading where they're the only kind we're supposed to eat, because of the sugar in regular potatoes."

Fowler, shaking his head, said, "What you're talking about is the glycemic index. And that's a topic that's largely misunderstood."

"Misunderstood because of the diet gurus who twist it into nonsense so they can sell books," Janice explained.

Fowler nodded in agreement. "According to the formula for calculating the glycemic index, you would have to eat a pound and a half of carrots before they register high on the index. Yet those diet books say to stay away from carrots, even though in the real world, the average serving of carrots is a small handful! The facts are twisted because they don't take practical serving sizes into account. And the same goes for white potatoes. Sure, sweet potatoes are more beneficial in terms of what's in them. They're also tasty and that's why we eat them on a regular basis. But give up white potatoes, possibly my favorite food, just for that? Ridiculous! All we have to do is keep a commonsense lid on portion sizes, and that means staying away from servings that can sink a ship, which is something we'll be talking about soon enough."

Janice said, "Facts can be manipulated and still not be

lies. That's how those people get away with it. But you can't manipulate real life and common sense!"

"Real life and common sense!" Fowler echoed, quickly dicing four large onions. "When I began developing the eight habits, that was the test they had to pass."

Karen nodded. She finished peeling the potatoes, cleaned them, then said, "Okay. Now what?"

"Now dice them, rinse them, and zap them in the microwave until they're soft. And while that's happening you can crack open—let's see, three for you, three for Janice and five for me—that's eleven eggs. Crack 'em. Use only three yolks and put them all into a large bowl."

Karen said, "You know, you can buy egg whites in cartons."

"That you can," Fowler said, giving the browning ground beef a good stir. "And it's an excellent choice, a real time-saver. I don't have any in the fridge today, but they're a regular on my shopping list." He moved from the stove to the cutting board and began to dice four celery stalks.

"Okay," Karen said, "eleven egg whites and three yolks, ready and waiting."

Fowler nodded. "Now put a drop of one-percent milk into them, a hefty splash of Tabasco, and beat those suckers. And watch what I'm going to do with this meat."

The ground beef was completely browned and sitting in an inch and a half of liquid fat. Fowler turned on the hot water, put a colander over the sink, and poured the meat into the colander, letting the fat drain while he filled the emptied pot with a couple of inches of water. He put the pot back onto the stove and set the burner on high. "Now I'm going to boil the meat for about two minutes," he said. "Then I'll drain it again, and when I'm finished there'll be practically no fat left. And I guarantee, when you taste the finished sauce you'll love it! Besides that, because of the amount I'm making, I've got a good ten spaghetti meals here, or two huge lasagnas. Or, if I spice it differently and mix in egg whites as a binder, I can use this meat to stuff a dozen green peppers or fill four shepherd's pies."

Karen stared at Fowler. "That's amazing. You've taken the worst of what's out there and turned it into the best! Lowfat meat sauce, lowfat lasagna, lowfat meat pies and stuffed peppers. Gary and I love that stuff!"

Fowler smiled. "I simply refuse to believe that any meal I want can't be made to be as low in fat as possible. I refuse to believe that it can't fit into the concepts of the habits. And when I start with that mind-set, plus a healthy dose of creativity, a good sense of humor—and no diet mentality—I always win."

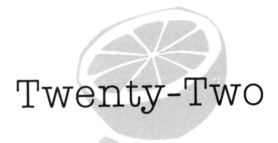

# Twenty-Two

"Okay," Fowler said to Karen, "the frying pans are in that cupboard."

Karen opened the cupboard he'd pointed out, and Fowler, talking quickly, said, "Let's start with one large pan for your spuds. Another smaller one for your omelet. Another for my turkey balls. And one more for Janice's omelet and then my scrambled eggs. And since we've already got the kettle on and the meat boiling, we're cooking the way I like to cook—like maniacs!"

Karen laughed.

"He's getting ready to blow," Janice said, smiling. "I've seen this before. It could be dangerous." She had given Gabe his pacifier and he was sitting quietly now, his bright dark eyes fixed on Janice.

"That's me," Fowler said. "Dangerous!" He snapped off the cover to the pump oil sprayer and, using only five pumps per pan, sprayed first one frying pan, then another, then another.

Janice said, "Go get 'em, killer!"

"Okay," Fowler said to Karen, "let's get those spuds going, and the green pepper and mushrooms and onions. And while you're doing that, I'll get the turkey smoking."

Working with a full smile and at an exaggerated pace, Fowler pulled two packages of ground turkey breast from the refrigerator, ripped open the packages and placed the meat into a bowl. Breaking up the meat with a fork, he said, "I just got another brainstorm! Listen to this." He turned to Janice, winked, then said to Karen, "We talked about creativity, right?"

"Right."

"Well, inside the habits there are really two kinds of creativity. The most important kind, the one we already talked about, says, within your comfort zone, you'll do whatever has to be done to follow the nutritional road map of the eight habits."

But before Fowler could continue, Karen asked, "Why do you always begin any discussion of the habits with the phrase *within your comfort zone?*"

Janice said, "He does that because that was the way he originally devised the habits. By first constructing the logic of the habit, understanding the need for it, then applying more and more effort to it while judging how it could become a part of his life, without *interfering* with his life. He used to call it his balancing act."

"That's right," Fowler said with a laugh. "My balancing act. You see, staying within your comfort zone is key, because if any part of any of the habits becomes irritating, then it becomes useless. Just like a diet."

Karen nodded. "So that's why we each create our own nutritional road map, right? Because we do it the way you did, by first understanding the reason for the habit, then by personalizing it to our individual needs and urges, the way . . .

well, the way you did with the sugar in your tea and the soy pepperoni."

"Exactly," Fowler replied. "And my road map, the way I bring the habits into my life, is not quite the same as Janice's. And yours will be different from either of ours."

"Okay . . . " Karen said. "And with the habits personalized, they then fit into each of our lives without being a struggle, the way diets are a struggle—because diets leave no room to maneuver."

"Exactly," Fowler said. "After a while you won't notice the habits, because they become so ingrained, so second nature, that they disappear."

"That's key too, isn't it?" Karen said. "After making the right choices, and after being prepared, it's a matter of sticking with the habits until they become second nature, become a positive new way of life, one that replaces all the old negative ways. It's got to become so ingrained that it disappears, the way it has for you. That's when it becomes an invisible part of your life—that's with you for the rest of your life. You don't even realize you're working with them anymore, do you? It's just become the way things are."

Fowler grinned. "That's exactly right. For us, they disappeared a long time ago."

"Along with your excess weight," Karen said. She shook her head wistfully, then added, "You were saying there are two kinds of creativity. So what's the other?"

"The other," Fowler answered, "is this." He opened the cupboard where he kept his herbs and spices and, with a flourish and a quick change back to overdrive, picked out the pepper, garlic powder, dried dill, sage, and Tabasco and Worcestershire sauces. While tossing single shakes of one and double shakes of another into the ground turkey, he said, "Have fun! Experiment! Don't be afraid! The only people who can't dance are the ones who won't get onto the dance floor!"

Then he suddenly stopped everything he was doing and,

furrowing his brow, asked Karen, "Are you sure you're crazy enough to be working in my kitchen?"

Karen, with a quick, sly expression of her own, answered, "I don't know. Why don't you test me?"

Janice, reaching for Gabe's hands, said excitedly, "Watch your mommy. After today she may never be the same!" Gabe screeched in delight. The pacifier popped from his mouth and Janice put it back in.

Fowler, his hands now wrist-deep in the turkey mix, said to Karen, "Okay. I don't want you to think. Just follow my instructions, one after the other, without taking a breath. And it's gonna be fast. Ready?"

"Ready!"

"Good." He raised one eyebrow, paused a full five seconds, then, like a drill sergeant barking orders, shouted, "Toss the spuds! Pour half of the egg mixture into the green pepper and mushrooms! Pour the rest into a bowl! Toss the spuds! Take the kettle off the burner! Toss the spuds! Throw the onions and celery into that pot! Mow the lawn! Toss the spuds!"

Karen kept up with Fowler's instructions until she got to the "mow the lawn" part. Then she threw her hands into the air and laughed at the all-out silliness she and Fowler and Janice were capable of. She looked at Janice, looked at Fowler and, with her face flushed red, laughed again, this time exploding into a howl so loud and full that Courage jumped to his feet with his hackles raised and began to bark.

Karen said to Fowler, "I'll mow the lawn and you pave the street and Janice and Gabe will discover new planets and Courage'll—"

The doorbell rang, followed immediately by pounding on the door. A deep, loud, furious voice yelled, "Karen! I know you're in there and I want you to get the hell out! Now!"

143

# Twenty-Three

Karen pushed her cart up the aisle of the grocery store. Inside the cart were two economy-sized packages of chips, two boxes of individually wrapped chocolate cakes, three two-liter bottles of cola, a dozen assorted frozen meals and a large tub of chocolate ice cream. She stopped the cart and put in two boxes of toaster pastries.

It was mid-afternoon. The store was crowded. Gabe, buckled into the cart's bright blue baby seat, had his fist around the plastic turnip Fowler had given him. The last time Karen had seen Fowler was eight days before, the morning Gary had appeared at Fowler's door and demanded that she come home.

She reached for a box of Sweet Smacks, feeling the heavy sway of fat beneath her arm. Suddenly her eyes met Fowler's. She held his stare for only an instant before quickly steering her cart away from his and around the corner.

At the end of this aisle she looked back to see if he had

followed her, but he hadn't. She pressed her jaws together, knowing this wasn't supposed to happen. A moment later she turned her cart back into the aisle to find him. When she saw him moving toward her, she waited.

"Hello," Fowler said.

"Don't you do this at night?" Karen asked. "I told myself I didn't have to worry about running into you."

"I changed my schedule."

"Just now? This week? After so many years?"

Fowler shrugged. "How are you?"

"I'm fine. Getting back to normal. The situation is working itself out. This last week has been quiet."

"We were worried about you."

"I know. I knew you would be. I'm sorry." In a muted tone she added, "Gary asked me not to see you again. Not to get in touch." All she could be, she knew, was honest. When she'd left Fowler's house, she'd gone in the only direction she saw ahead of her, back to the security of hopelessness. She struggled to keep that emotion out of her voice.

Fowler touched her arm. "Why does he keep saying that?"

Karen sighed. "He doesn't like it when I'm with other people. He's always been that way—protective. And now, with the baby . . . "

"He has a strange way of being protective," Fowler replied, his voice neutral.

Karen moved her cart to the side and said quietly, "Fowler, sometimes things happen in a marriage that look one way on the outside and another on the inside. Gary is suspicious by nature; I knew that when I married him. He's suspicious and jealous and very private. So he was upset when I met you. You know that. He understood how it happened, though. He just wasn't happy about it. And then when I told him about the things you were teaching me— you know, about nutrition, about the Power of One Good Habit—it bothered him even more."

"How could learning about nutrition bother him?"

Karen smiled sheepishly. "You're not a doctor, Fowler. But Gary says you think you are. He says you're acting like some mystical know-it-all and thinks there might be more to what you're doing than just being helpful. He's worried you're trying to take over my mind, turn me into some sort of follower, like they do in cults. He thinks you might be dangerous."

She knew Fowler could tell she didn't believe a word Gary had said. She went on, though. "He also said that if there was anything wrong with any of the food in this store, they wouldn't be able to sell it."

"Well," Fowler answered her, "at least there, on a certain level, he's right."

"He is?"

"Of course. There's no food in this store that could be labeled poison. No warning on anything that says, 'Eat too much of this and you'll eventually get blocked arteries or diabetes or cancer and die.'" He paused, and then asked, "What about your weight? Did you tell him the Power of One Good Habit would help with that?"

Karen nodded.

"And?"

"When it comes to my weight, Gary only believes one thing—that it's because I'm lazy."

Fowler's expression remained blank.

Karen continued, "He said I should get an abs machine, the kind they advertise on TV." She smiled wryly. "He tried to get me to do some sit-ups last night. He was holding my feet, but I couldn't do even one. I couldn't lift myself off the ground."

"What did he say about that?"

"The usual."

Fowler reached out to Gabe, saying, "Hey, little guy. How're you doing?" But Gabe was more interested in the wall of brightly colored boxes than in Fowler. Fowler said to Karen, "What about *Gary's* weight? How's that?"

"He's big," Karen answered, "like me. Maybe sixty

pounds overweight. But it's different on a man. Gary says women like their men big, that it gives them a sense of security." Once more she shrugged her shoulders, then added, "Fowler, I know he's not perfect, but I need Gary for a lot of reasons. So does Gabe. He's a wonderful father, and beneath all his anger, he's really a good man. And in his own way, he loves me. I know that."

"I'm glad he does," Fowler replied, glancing at the items in Karen's cart.

Karen, watching him, said, "That's why I didn't want you to see me. I didn't want you to know what I was buying."

"Why not? Gary says all this is fine, otherwise they wouldn't be allowed to sell it."

In a very soft voice, Karen said, "I know he's wrong. And I know you're right. And I know everything about the habits is right. But, Fowler, there are all kinds of people in this world, and some people, like me . . . we're the kind who just can't . . . " She paused.

"Can't what?" Fowler pressed. "Can't make the habits work?"

"That's right. I'm one of those people it won't work for. I know that from my own history. Any kind of success with losing weight passes me by. And I've learned to accept that. Maybe Gary knows what he's talking about. Maybe when it comes to losing weight, I just don't get it."

Fowler reached into Karen's cart and lifted out the tub of chocolate ice cream and said, "Tell me about this. What's in it?"

"Fat," Karen answered quickly, having thought about it long before Fowler asked the question.

"And?"

"And sugar, lots of it. And the fat and sugar make it taste good." She'd thought about that, too. Used that obvious truth to get it from the grocery-store freezer into her cart.

"That's right," Fowler said. "It does taste good. And I also love ice cream, and I eat it regularly. But even though it tastes good, how did you feel when you put it into your cart?"

"Lousy," Karen admitted, shaking her head. "Weak and angry."

"Why did you feel that way?"

"Because I know it's garbage. And this is garbage too," she added, pointing to the chips. "And so are the drinks and the frozen meals. None of it fits into the concepts of the habits."

"Then it's working," Fowler said.

"What?"

"It's working. The Power of One Good Habit is working. The knowledge of the battle is in you now, and that knowledge has gotten to you. The fact of the war has gotten to you. It's gone from your brain to your emotions. You can feel the fight and you can feel your loss of control. And there's nothing you can do to stop that." He took a deep breath. "You can still buy this kind of food, and eat it. But you can never be the same with it. In fact, you can never really enjoy it again, not until you know all eight habits, not until you can slot even *this* food comfortably into the habit it belongs to— until you can eat it, the way I do, knowing all you have to know. And then you'll savor it, I guarantee. But not until then."

Karen found herself staring at him.

Fowler smiled. "Just the knowledge of it, just knowing the fact of the war, has already changed your life."

Karen, her voice barely a whisper, said, "It *has* changed my life. There were times during this past week when I wasn't sure whether it was knowing what they, the manufacturers of this junk, are doing to me, that got me so mad, or if it was you. The fact that you opened my eyes to it, that was upsetting me. But what I know for sure is that I can't stop reciting the first four habits as though they were a mantra. I see them in my mind like your neon sign. Find the fats. Include breakfast. Tame my sweet tooth. Replace processed and chemically enhanced foods with wholesome close-to-the-farm foods. And do all of it within my comfort zone. Without feeling any of my diet guilt or frustrations."

She looked away from him for a moment. She looked at

Gabe, who was playing with his turnip again. Then she said quickly, "Because of you I know it's me against them. The enemy. I know that. And I know that the enemy is getting rich at the same time that it's slowly but surely killing me. Now when I drive down the street and see the fast-food places or hear food ads on the radio or see them on TV, I think: You're out to get me! You've turned making me fat into advertising science. Moneymaking science. You're destroying my health and my family's health for the sake of a buck!"

She looked directly at Fowler. "And it was you who did this to me. You and Janice opened my eyes. A couple of weeks ago I would have bought this ice cream and felt as though I was buying comfort. Even excitement. Taking home a friend. Now I buy it and I know I'm letting the enemy into my house . . . I feel like a traitor!"

"Traitor?" Fowler said, his eyes widening. "That's perfect! That's the perfect word, the perfect description." Then he added, "Traitor to whom, though?"

"To me?" Karen asked hesitantly.

Fowler smiled. He touched Karen on the arm and said, "Do you have time for a coffee?"

# Twenty-Four

Though she spoke to them twice on the telephone, the first chance Karen had to see Fowler and Janice again was eight days after meeting Fowler in the grocery store. This time she drove to their house, with Gabe strapped into his child seat behind her. On the way over, she thought, *For once, at least, they're in for a pleasant surprise.*

She was smiling when Janice opened the front door.

Janice stared. For a moment she forgot to back her wheel-chair away from the open door so no one passing by could see her.

Wearing gardening gloves and carrying a spade, Fowler came up behind Karen, saying, "I saw you drive up." When she turned to face him he reacted with a single word. "Wow!"

She was dressed in a printed skirt and white blouse and blue jacket. Her hair, newly trimmed and tinted, was now shorter, tighter to her face and more appealing. She had put on makeup and her nails were polished. But most of all there was a new air about her.

"You're glowing," Janice said approvingly. "As though you're being lit from within."

"Thank you," Karen replied. "I feel that way—lit from within."

"I'd say it looks more like you won the lottery," Fowler said.

"To a certain extent I have," Karen answered. "But this lottery has nothing to do with money, and everything to do with life."

"Well, come on in!" Janice said.

Fowler left his spade and gloves and boots by the front door. He reached for Gabe, who went happily into his arms.

In the kitchen Fowler placed Gabe into his seat. Then he went behind the counter and returned with three glasses of water with lemon and his container of precut vegetables with dip. He moved the large fruit bowl to the side, and Janice's pad and pen closer to her.

Janice, touching Gabe's foot, shaking it lightly, said to Karen, "What did you mean when you said you won a lottery that has nothing to do with money and everything to do with life?"

"Well," Karen answered, taking off Gabe's sweater, "you probably know that I met Fowler at the grocery store."

Janice nodded.

"And that he told me the greatest change in his life occurred when he finally realized that everything he was learning was useless, until he tied it to the power of choice. He said that it's only when we begin to make those choices that the changes in our life begin." She gave Gabe his pacifier and taking her seat, added, "Then he showed me how choices are everywhere, not just on the grocery shelves, but even in how we think about ourselves, even think about others."

"You didn't tell me that," Janice said to her father.

Fowler shrugged and turned to Karen. "All I told Janice was that the two of us went through the store a second time and picked out replacements for the food in your basket. I thought I'd leave anything else for you to say, if you wanted."

"Thank you," Karen said. Then to Janice, she added, "It's all about choices. I see that now. What to wear in the morning, what to eat, even how to view the day. Once the realization is there, that the choice is ours, truly ours alone, and that we can literally choose to either move forward or stay behind, the power of choice becomes . . . liberating."

"Knowledge is power and we all have choices," Fowler said softly.

Janice smiled at her father. She said to Karen, "He taught me about choices too, showed me I had the choice to fall back on my disability or go beyond it. That all it took was one step, a tiny step that I had to make in my mind. And in an instant I went from *I can't* to *I can*. For me, that's when everything changed."

Fowler said, "The biggest challenge is getting past the roadblocks in our own minds."

Karen was nodding. "And doing that gets easier with practice. All week I've been saying to myself, I have a choice in everything. And the ability to choose makes me powerful. For the first time in my life *I* feel in control!" She laughed. "In just a few weeks, between learning about the Power of One Good Habit and understanding the power of choice, the two of you have given me more to think about than I've had to think through in my entire thirty-two years."

"If we helped, then I'm pleased," Fowler said.

Janice was beaming.

"You helped, all right," Karen said. "And you're still helping." She reached into the baby tote bag and took out her journal. "My first choice was that I'm going to take control of my life—move it, without telling Gary, from his hands to mine. And at the same time, work on our marriage. It's a big order, I know. But I think I can do it. I think I can focus on both my family and myself, together. And part of focusing on myself is choosing my own friends and deciding what's important to me. And I want the two of you as friends, even if, for a while at least, it's better for me not to tell that to Gary."

"Those aren't just some small adjustments to your life, they're major changes," Janice said. "Don't you think that sooner or later Gary's going to find out?"

"Yes. He will. In fact, I'm planning on telling him myself. Just not quite yet. You see, as part of choosing to work on my marriage, of making it better, I'll only tell Gary about the habits at a time when telling him won't turn into an argument. I want my telling him to be positive, for both of us. And I'm laying the groundwork for that now, not just hoping it'll happen."

She took a long drink from the glass of water in front of her, then smiled. "In the last week or so, since realizing the *choice* is mine, I've become exceptionally good to Gary—you know, caring and loving. And frankly, at the moment, I don't think he knows what to make of it! He's been quiet. I think he's trying to understand."

Fowler said, "It's hard to challenge a change that obviously makes life better. No one can easily start an argument over 'Why are you being so good to me?'"

"That's exactly it!" Karen said. "It is better now. More peaceful, anyway. I keep telling myself it's all about choices, and I'm the one doing the choosing. And the next thing I say is, Okay, what choice can I make today, now, this minute, to make our marriage better? And then I do it, something, anything, even if it's just a kiss on the cheek." She laughed lightly. "The poor guy is perplexed by all of it, by my new attitude toward him and my attitude toward myself. And all he's seen so far is what shows on the surface. When it comes to me, right now, most of the changes are happening beneath my skin . . . "

She paused. "Go on," Fowler said. "You can't make a statement like that and stop there!"

Karen said, "I've decided to make the Power of One Good Habit a permanent part of our lives, whether Gary knows it or not." She held up her journal. "I want to understand each of the habits, then begin applying them to my life the same way you did when you first developed them, by working with each one slowly, letting it adapt to me while I adapt to it. I want to maintain my comfort level while my excitement grows, with no diet anxieties, none of that diet mentality that I hate."

She took another sip of water. Then, with her words tumbling through a laugh, said, "I've started it already, even though I only know the first four habits. And in just the first week I've lost two and a half pounds! This is the first time I've ever lost weight without being on a diet, by *eating* my weight off, and I feel unbelievably wonderful! Even my friend Sue, from work, noticed the change. Yesterday she stopped by my desk and said I looked great and there was something different about me. She saw me eating a meal I brought from home, something I've never done before. So I told her about the Power of One Good Habit, all that I know so far, especially that it's not a diet—and now she wants to try it, too!"

Fowler laughed.

Janice said, "I'm not surprised. That's the power of common sense."

"Common sense and real life!" Fowler said. He reached for the vegetable platter.

Karen said, "Of course Gary doesn't know what I'm doing, because when it comes to the food in our house, that's all left up to me." She laughed again. "Gary's living with the first four habits, at least at home, and he doesn't even know it! It's that subtle, so unlike any diet I've ever been on. Even the fruit! It's there now, on the coffee table *and* the kitchen counter. I keep both bowls full. And that's all it takes."

Fowler, smiling, said, "It's because it's there, staring at you."

"It's true!" Karen said. "We've both been eating at least three pieces a day—just because it looks so tempting. And you were right: my sweet tooth's just about gone! I didn't believe it could happen, but it works!" She pointed to the vegetables and dip on the table. "I've even caught Gary snacking on the cut-up veggies with dip that I keep in a container in the fridge. You're right there too. It's because it's there. That's the key. Now when we look in the fridge to see what to eat, we snack. The veggies have become our thinking-about-what-to-eat snack. And for me it's my eating-while-I-cook snack."

She shook the journal in Fowler's direction. "Now I want to know what I'm missing. I want to learn the last four habits." But before Fowler could say anything, she added, lowering her voice, "First, though, I have a confession to make. This past week, another thing I realized was that when I first told you I wanted to learn about the eight habits, that I'd found the necessary courage to do that, I was wrong."

"How could you have been wrong?" Janice asked. "That's exactly what you said—I want to learn the eight habits. How could you say that and not have the courage to do it?"

Karen shook her head. "Because that's what we do. That's what overweight people do. We lie to ourselves about courage."

Fowler nodded.

Karen caught Fowler's expression and said, "You knew what was happening, didn't you? You knew I was lying to myself about making an honest attempt at controlling my weight."

"I am you," Fowler replied gently.

"I don't understand," Janice said. "How could you have been lying to yourself?"

Karen sighed. "The lie. It's how we overweight people protect ourselves, what we project to the world. It's the mask between what we *wish* we could do and what we *believe* we can do. We say we will lose the weight, but in our hearts know we won't. So we don't even try. We just lie about it, lie about the effort to ourselves and to others, sometimes knowingly and sometimes unknowingly. And then we fail."

Fowler, looking at Janice, said, "What we do is attempt to

try, but don't attempt to succeed. And so we don't. We sabotage our efforts, pretend the sabotage is not there, and then fail, saying, 'I tried, but for me, for some reason, it just didn't work.' Then we walk away until the next time."

"That's it exactly," Karen whispered.

For a long moment there was silence.

Karen lifted her glass of water to her lips and took several slow swallows, then put the glass back on the table.

"I don't know if there's anything more simple to describe, and more complicated to accomplish, than losing weight," Fowler said. "It's true that for some people, being overweight might be a medical problem, and they might need medical help. And for others it could be a psychological problem, perhaps a childhood trauma that's at the root of it, and they need help to recover from that. But for most of us, most of the nation, the problem of being overweight comes from only one source."

Fowler smiled, and then, in a booming, announcer-style voice he said, "Attention! Attention, every overweight person on the planet! Eat less—and you'll lose weight." Then he solemnly dipped his head, pretending to bow, and said, "Thank you."

Karen said, "The Power of One Good Habit will do exactly that!"

"Yes, it will," Fowler agreed. "But it's not a magic pill. You can't try to lift that glass of water. You can only lift it."

Karen looked at Fowler, then at the glass of water in front of her. She put her fingers around it and, after a long, reflective pause, lifted it. And with the glass aloft, she slowly said, "You're right. I can't *try* to lift the glass. I can only lift it. And I can't *try* to live the eight habits. I can only live them."

"That's the only way," Fowler said. "You can't try it. It's not a change of clothing. It's not something that can be tried on, checked for its fit, then tossed and forgotten. Once the knowledge is in you, once you understand why you're overweight, who the enemy is and how each of the habits works, you can only live it, or with your knowledge and consent, ignore it. But you can't try it for a while or fail at it over time. It's not a piece of clothing or an exam, not something that has an end."

"Live it, or knowingly ignore it," Karen repeated.

Fowler nodded. "Okay, enough of this seriousness." He lifted his glass of water, took a good swallow and, tilting the glass in Karen's direction, said, "Are you ready to learn the next habit?"

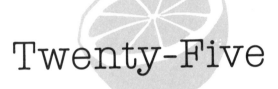

# Twenty-Five

Fowler turned to Janice. "And Habit Number Five is?" he asked.

"Water."

"Water?" Karen said.

"That's it," Fowler said. "A one-word habit that means so much I don't know where to begin explaining it."

"Believe it or not," Janice said, "this is the habit that took him the longest to figure out."

"But I've heard about this one before," Karen said, reaching under Gabe's arm for his pacifier and putting it back into his mouth. "We're supposed to drink water, right? A certain amount of water? Eight glasses, I think."

Fowler was nodding. "If you have to put a number on it, then eight is as good as any. That's the number that's always bandied about. And that's the number I also work around. But remember, I'm not counting anything—not calories or grams or pounds or glasses of water or anything."

Janice said, "In fact, there is no exact right amount when it comes to daily water consumption, because factors like exercise, temperature, age and body size all play a part."

"That's true," Fowler said, "but as one of the eight habits, it's also beside the point. Because just like all the other habits, nothing about this one is set in stone. If one day I drink six eight-ounce glasses of water and the next day eleven, then that's what it is. This habit, like all the rest, has to fit into my life, and not the other way around." He smiled as though he was holding back a secret, and then lifted his glass into the air. "Let me tell you about water. The little I know."

In a mock whisper, Janice said to Karen, "He knows it all. Probably more than the so-called experts."

"I know," Karen said. "I've thought about that. It's because he's living it, walking the walk."

"Water," Fowler said, seemingly oblivious to their exchange, "is our body's most important nutrient, for a whole slew of scientific reasons, none of which I'm going to go into. Instead, what I'm going to do is go back to the image of my old clunker. And in that car, if carbohydrates are the fuel, then water is an internal carwash. It's a cleaning agent with a miraculous kick, one that's able to not only flush out everything that needs to be flushed, but also power the reaction, the way oxygen powers fire. Water takes care of our insides and outsides, our internal organs and our skin. Water, plain old water, is one of the keys to turning that clunker into a hot new Ferrari."

"Just water?" Karen asked.

"Just water. Plain old water, except with that twist of lemon I love, or a splash of lime. But water. Nothing with sugar or caffeine."

"So all I have to do is drink water?" Karen asked.

Fowler nodded. "That's all you have to do. But don't be fooled by how simple it seems, because it's not."

Janice said, "That's what happened to him at the

beginning. He just said, I have to drink water, then forgot about it and went on with the other habits."

"It's because it seems so easy," Fowler said. "I just accepted it, then basically ignored it, sort of shrugged it into my life without digging deeper. I didn't bother to focus on it the way I did with the other habits."

"Tell her what happened," Janice said, smiling at Gabe who had reached out to her. She gave him her index finger and he clutched it and began babbling softly.

Fowler said to Karen, "I'd gotten all the other habits down pat. After years of hit-and-miss. Of experimenting. Of highs and lows and then of going wild with creativity, I'd reached the point where I was comfortable with my degree of focus and participation in all the other habits. I didn't have to *think* about them anymore. I was living them to the point where they'd grown invisible."

"Except for the water," Janice said.

"That's right. Except for this concept of drinking water, I was living the habits. And the effect of seeing my results, and letting the excitement that came from those results push me into working for even greater results, had been pounding away at me so much that I'd already regained my health and lost most of my extra weight. For me, at that point, my weight was where I figured it would stay. And I was more than just pleased with it—I was thrilled!"

Karen nodded. She could only imagine how thrilling that would be.

"But I'd never focused on the water," Fowler continued. "I just drank it when I was thirsty and ignored it the rest of the time. Then I began to think about it and I wondered: just how much water is eight glasses? And what does it mean to actually drink that much? So I filled an eight-glass pitcher of water and in just one day realized, Hey, this is a *lot* of water! And I'm having a lot of trouble getting it all down!" He paused. "So I focused."

"He became creative," Janice said.

"That's right. I knew I liked the taste of lemon, so I began

160

with that. I put a slice of lemon into my glass. And that was better. For me, it was actually *much* better. Then, to make things even simpler, I began using lemon juice from a jar, or crystallized lemon from an envelope, mixing that into my bottle or pitcher filled with water, and keeping the pitcher close at hand." He smiled. "But I still wasn't drinking eight glasses. Not easily. Not at a level I found comfortable."

"It's because he still had to *think* about it," Janice said. "And he likes to have everything about the eight habits just flow, become a seamless part of his world so he can ignore them and get on with the rest of his life."

"That's right. And it was bothering me, because it seems so simple. So I focused harder and I thought: How would it be if I *began* my day with water? What if I started out with my pitcher of cold, lemon-flavored water? So I tried it. And I found that the taste of the lemon, first thing in the morning, completely changed the water into a drink that I found not just tasty, but also cleansing. It had the effect of cleaning my palate, as if preparing it for the new day. And I liked that."

"He used to describe it as a second mouthwash," Janice said. "One that went all the way to the back of his throat and then down to his stomach."

"It did feel that way, and it still does! And when I started drinking it first thing in the morning, I had no trouble drinking eight glasses. In fact, I found myself often refilling my eight-glass pitcher by noon! And by also keeping a bottle of water in my car and carrying around another with me in the garden, by the end of the day I might have had twelve or thirteen or more glasses. All without trouble. Without a thought. All within my comfort level. But remember, except for that time while I was focusing on the habit, experimenting with it, deciding how to best tailor it to fit my needs and my life, I don't count glasses."

"Tell her the rest," Janice said impatiently.

Fowler said, "What I also discovered—"

"He was amazed," Janice interrupted.

"Yes, I was truly amazed. Because after figuring out how

to apply this habit to my life, I found that those last few extra pounds I was carrying, pounds I was fully and happily prepared to live with, also started to come off."

"Those extra pounds came off just by drinking more water?" Karen asked.

"Yes! Within weeks of drinking my lemon-flavored, eye-opening, palate-cleansing, first-thing-in-the-morning, then-for-the-rest-of-the-day-sipping water, the extra pounds began to melt away. Pound after pound, week after week, until they were gone. Just *gone!*" He grinned.

"But it wasn't the water by itself," Janice said.

"No! Don't get me wrong, Karen. Water by itself won't cause weight loss. But it's a necessary *addition* to all the other habits. It gives them the extra boost they need." Fowler grinned again and shrugged. "Really, until I tried it, I never even suspected there was anything else I could do with the Power of One Good Habit that would impress me. But there was. And it was the addition of water."

He lifted his glass to Karen. "To this simplest, most logical of habits—good old water. It's truly astounding."

Karen was smiling. "To water!" she echoed, raising her glass. She took a good swallow then put her glass down, still smiling.

Janice narrowed her eyes. "What is it? What are you smiling at? It's like you have a secret."

"I do," Karen said. "Even without you telling me about this habit, I've begun drinking water with lemon. Having it here with you, sipping it constantly, started to get me . . . used to it. Even more than used to it: liking it! Liking that cleansing taste you talked about. The best part of it for me though, is that it's begun moving me away from my own *worst* habit: drinking those sodas all day."

Fowler was nodding.

Janice said, "There's nothing worse than sodas and all those other sugar- and calorie-filled drinks out there!" She sounded disgusted. "Do you know that just one twelve-ounce can of soda or punch a day can double your chances of getting type-two diabetes?"

"I didn't know that," Karen said. "How come that isn't on the labels? It should be!"

"What's not written doesn't constitute a lie," Janice said. "Though there are health organizations that are lobbying hard to make this kind of information mandatory." She did a quick calculation on her pad, then said to Karen, "How many pounds do you think you'd lose in a year if you drank thirty-two ounces of water with lemon every day instead of that same amount of soda?"

Karen shook her head. "I know it's a lot . . . Ten, at least. Maybe fifteen."

"Not even close."

"Twenty?"

"Forty-five."

"No way!" Karen was amazed.

Janice nodded, smiling. "That's right. By replacing your daily liter of soda with water and lemon, you'll lose forty-five pounds in the next year."

"But that's almost all I have to lose."

Fowler said, "If I could get everyone in the country to do just one thing for their weight and health, it would be that: exchange their sugar-filled drinks for water with lemon."

Janice looked at Karen and said, "Water with lemon. Now that's the Power of One Good Habit!"

# Twenty-Six

"All right," Fowler said. "We've done enough talking about water. It's time to *eat*!" But instead of getting up and going to the cooking area, he leaned casually back in his chair, crossed his arms over his chest, looked Karen in the eye and, after a moment's pause, said to her, "Before we eat, though, I have an important question to ask you."

"Okay?"

"Are you hungry?"

"Am I hungry? Me?" She gestured toward herself with her thumb and grinned. "Of course I'm hungry! I'm always hungry. I'm always *starving*!"

"Good," Fowler replied. "That's good. What's *not* so good is that today is one of my lazy days. In fact, right now I'm so lazy I don't even want to get out of my chair. But I still want a great meal, one that follows all the habits, and I want it now!"

Janice smiled. Karen said to her, "It sounds as though he's setting me up for something."

"I am," Fowler replied. "You're still my *sous-chef*, right?"

"Yes, sir, mister, sir," Karen answered, saluting.

"Good. Then I want you to go to the freezer and await further instructions."

Karen, wearing a quizzical grin, stood and headed for the cooking area. As soon as she stood, Gabe reached out his hands for her, emitted a tentative, questioning sound, then began to cry.

"Oh no!" Janice said, reaching to reassure him. "She's not going away, sweetie!"

Karen quickly stepped back to the table. "It's not just me that he wants," she said, unbuckling Gabe and picking him up. "It's lunch." She rocked the baby, quickly calming him, and looked at Janice, "Would you mind? I have a date with the freezer."

"I'd love to!" Janice said.

Karen kissed Gabe and put him back into the baby seat, then took two small jars of baby food, a plastic spoon, a spill-proof baby cup, and a package of towelettes from her tote bag. "There, all set," she said, moving Gabe closer to Janice.

Janice picked up one of the bottles of food, read, "Mixed cereal with apple and banana," opened it, and, saying "Yummy!" to Gabe, began to feed him as though she'd been doing it since he was born.

Karen smiled at Fowler and shrugged. "Guess they don't need me."

"You've become irrelevant, so you may as well get to work in the kitchen."

Karen laughed, saluted again, then stepped behind the counter and opened the freezer door.

"Okay," Fowler said. "You can see that everything in there is labeled, so we know what it is. Now what I want from you is to pick out a smorgasbord of tastes for our lunch. A bit of everything."

"A bit of everything," Karen repeated, staring into the

freezer. But before taking anything out she turned to Fowler and said, "You know, what I'd love, one day, when you have the time, is a recipe for all of these. For everything that's in the freezer."

"Recipes?" Fowler said, standing. "That's easily solved." He pulled a tattered book from the shelf and propped it on its self-standing easel. "Here're my recipes: *Lickety-Split Meals For Health Conscious People on the Go.* I've been relying on this countertop coach for years, and by now I can practically recite everything that's in it. And not just the recipes, but the entire cooking philosophy. This book fits the Power of One Good Habit like a glove. It even tells you how to stock your pantry. So you can have it. Temporarily. Until you get your own. Because this copy has all my favorite stains."

"Thank you!" Karen exclaimed, picking up the worn and earmarked book, eager to uncover the magic behind Fowler's restaurant.

But before she could glance through it, Fowler said, "Now, though, is not the time to begin reading, because I'm hungry, and so is Janice. And you're *starving*. Right? Wasn't that the word you used?"

"You'd better believe it," Karen said, setting the book down. "Okay," she said, turning back to the freezer. "You want a bit of everything. A tasting tray."

"Exactly," Fowler said. "A tasting tray for three."

Karen reached into the freezer, took out four packages and, reading the labels, said, "Okay, we'll start with a slice of Turkey Loaf, one Salmon Burger and a couple of packages of Un-fried Rice."

"Find the Creamy Chicken Enchiladas," Janice said to her, wiping a spill from Gabe's chin. "They're fantastic. You've got to have one with me."

"You can also take out some of the Un-stuffed Peppers and Hearty Bean and Pasta Stew," Fowler added. "The peppers are made with brown rice and the stew with whole-wheat pasta, and they're also both amazing."

"Creamy Chicken Enchiladas . . . Un-stuffed Peppers . . .

Hearty Bean and Pasta Stew . . . " Karen read out loud, as one by one she took the packages from the freezer.

"And don't forget the vegetables," Fowler reminded her. "I want to see a yellow one and an orange one and at least two shades of green."

"Okay, okay!" Karen said, laughing. She reached in and took out a package of frozen vegetables. "That's more than enough! We've got a meal here fit for royalty."

Moving around the kitchen as though she'd been raised in it, Karen found two large microwaveable containers and placed the Turkey Loaf, Salmon Burger and Un-fried Rice in one container, and the Creamy Chicken Enchiladas and Un-stuffed Peppers into the other. She put both containers, plus the container of Hearty Bean and Pasta Stew, into the microwave, set the timer and pressed start. Next she took out a large pot and steamer, poured in a triple serving of the frozen mixed vegetables and got that going.

Janice said, "You know, I didn't realize how hungry I was. Just hearing that list of food has gotten my juices flowing."

"I can hardly believe it," Karen said. "One incredible meal, coming up in a matter of minutes. Even if we ordered in, it would take longer than that." She thought about it for a moment, then said, "It's all about preparation. As basic as that. About taking advantage of your energy when you have it, and saving it."

Fowler said, "Now all we need is more water."

"Oops. The water. Coming right up." Karen refilled the glasses. "What's next, boss?"

"Next," Fowler replied, "I want you to tell me you're still starving."

Karen laughed. "Of course I'm still starving! I'm always starving. Starving is a part of me, like an extra leg, like the horns on a great big moose! It goes where I go, does what I do. It leads the way and leads my life!"

"We already told you, though, that a healthy appetite is a sign of good health."

"Then I am one unbelievably healthy—and heavy—"

167

"I'm also hungry," Janice said, cutting in.

"Hungry? Or starving?" Karen wanted to know.

"Just hungry."

"What about you?" Karen said to Fowler. "Are you hungry, or starving?"

Fowler said, "I also have a healthy appetite. And I'm also hungry. In fact, at this moment I'm very hungry. But starving? No. And we'll talk about that, about your starving. But not now. Now I want to eat. And," he said, as the microwave began to beep, "suddenly I've got a ton of energy, so I'll serve the meal." He stood and motioned for Karen to take her seat. But before he went behind the counter, he stopped for a moment to look at Janice and Gabe. Shaking his head, he said, "You know, that's a sight I never thought I'd see."

"Me neither," Janice said, looking up at him and smiling.

For another few moments Fowler watched his daughter feed the baby, then he stepped behind the counter. There he took down a serving platter from one cupboard, and two plates from another, and lined up the three dishes side by side. Next he took the steaming-hot food from the microwave and onto the serving platter placed the slice of turkey loaf, the salmon burger, one of the enchiladas, a good cupful of Unfried Rice and a heaping quantity of the mixed vegetables. Then he poured a ladle of Hearty Bean and Pasta Stew into two serving bowls.

At the table, Janice said to Karen, "I think that's it. He doesn't want anymore."

Karen opened the second jar, saying to Gabe, "How about dessert?" She offered him a spoonful. The baby turned his head from this spoon too. "No? Okay, enough for now." Karen cleaned Gabe's chin and cheeks and hands with a towelette, saying to Janice, "I learned a lesson from my mother! Now I do the exact opposite of what she used to do; I don't force food on Gabe."

"No! Never do that!" Janice said quickly. "That archaic behavior should have been outlawed years ago. What we want to do is teach our children that it's *okay* to say, 'that's it, I've had enough.' "

Behind the counter, Fowler continued to prepare lunch. He put one of the enchiladas, a serving of the Unfried Rice and a cup of mixed vegetables on one of the plates. And on the other he placed the Unstuffed Peppers and a good serving of the mixed vegetables. Then he turned to Karen and Janice and said, "I'm ready here. How's it going there?"

"All ready," Karen said, putting the baby supplies back into her diaper bag.

Janice said to her, "He actually looks happier now. I mean . . . his expression. Like someone who was hungry and now he's not. Now he's perfectly comfortable."

Karen nodded. "It's already all there, even at this age. The personality, the expressions, what he likes to eat and what he doesn't. And especially who he likes and who he doesn't. It's already in that tiny package."

"It's really so amazing," Janice said, reaching for Gabe's hand.

Karen put Gabe's pacifier into his mouth.

Fowler brought the cutlery and napkins to the table, placed them around, then went back to the counter and returned with the two plates. He served the enchilada and Unfried Rice to Janice, and put the plate with the Unstuffed Peppers and a small bowl of Hearty Bean and Pasta Stew in front of his chair. Returning to the counter, he brought out the serving platter filled with enough food for three people, plus the second bowl of Hearty Bean and Pasta Stew, and placed them in front of Karen.

Karen stared at the huge amount of food in front of her, looked at Fowler and laughed uneasily.

Fowler said, "I hope everything's all right? You did say you were starving, didn't you?"

"Yes."

"And that you're always starving?"

"Yes!"

"Well, if you're always starving, you should be able to eat

169

continually. So it seems to me I might even have to refill this platter. Maybe several times."

"Fowler," Karen said. "You're making fun of—"

"I understand starving," Fowler cut in. "I saw the movie. And I don't want that to happen here, not in front of me, not in my restaurant. So let's eat, because Janice and I are both hungry. I have another habit to tell you about. And if you thought drinking water was one of the easiest, then this next one is definitely the hardest."

Karen sighed. She said to Gabe, "They want to make me fatter—after I've just lost two and a half pounds!" She shook her head in mock resignation. "But you know what? This smells too good to pass up! And at the moment I don't care about losing weight or gaining weight or anything else. I'm going to pretend that I'm alone and just eat."

"We'll talk about that, too," Fowler said, digging into his meal.

Karen said, "You know, this meat loaf—"

"Turkey," Janice corrected.

"Right, turkey loaf—it's really unbelievable. I don't think I've ever tasted anything quite like it before."

"And you probably won't again," Janice said.

Karen, her mouth full, managed to ask, "Why not?" She finished her bite of turkey loaf, took a bite of the salmon burger and said, "Wow! This is really excellent too!"

"I'll tell you why you won't taste what you're eating now again," Janice answered. "Do you remember what my father told us about creativity with the habits? That within the concepts of the habits there are really two types of creativity— the creativity he uses to tailor each of the habits to his life, the way he did by putting lemon in his water or using the soy pepperoni for his pizza, or finding the fat or sugar in a meal and reducing it to as low as possible."

"That part's a game," Fowler said. "I still have fun with it."

"It's *all* a game to you," Janice said to her father. "All eight habits. You have fun with them all!"

"You're right. I do have fun with them. I know I'm not supposed to, but I do. I like making them easy, making them . . . invisible. And I like the results."

Janice, still looking at her father, said, "You know, you shouldn't be saying that. According to all the overweight people out there, you're supposed to be struggling with this, moaning about all the good stuff you're not allowed to eat and how you'll never be able to make it last, not spending the last ten years having fun." She smiled and shook her head, then turned to Karen. "Where was I? Oh, yes: creativity. There's the tailoring part of it: making the habits easy, even fun. Then there's this," she said, pointing to her Un-fried Rice. "The going-wild-in-the-kitchen side. And when it comes to this creativity, there's less to it than meets the eye."

"Less than meets the eye? What do you mean?" Karen asked.

"What I mean is that if my father can cook like this, then anyone can! He might be a genius at taking nutritional complexities and reducing them into simple guidelines, simple habits. But when it comes to cooking, to this part of it, the flavor part—"

"Okay, okay," Fowler said. "If we're going to air my kitchen secrets, then at least let me do the airing." He looked at Karen. "It goes like this: let's say there's a sale at the grocery store on peppers, so naturally I buy a few . . . "

"Twenty," Janice supplied, lightly caressing Gabe's arm.

"All right, twenty. Enough for the entire platoon. Then with all those peppers I say, well, I just happen to have all this cooked brown rice in the fridge."

"About a ton of it," Janice said. "He likes to make his big batches of anything in stages, spread over a few days, so he doesn't really do very much at one time."

Fowler shrugged. "My concentration span is limited, and like everyone else, so is my time." He grinned, then said, "Where was I? Oh, yes: the peppers. So I snoop around the kitchen a bit more and I find some garlic, some onions, some carrots and tomatoes."

"But the flavor?" Karen asked, thinking, *Spread out the work, that's an idea I can use. Buy a lot at one time and make a big batch, then store it as individual meals in the freezer like Fowler.*

"The flavor," Fowler said, "is what I do when I've got the basics covered—I go for it." He grinned. "Janice is right: in this restaurant you'll never taste exactly the same thing twice, because the flavor you're tasting now belongs to anything I might have had in the kitchen at the time I made it. It could be any combination of oregano or garlic or thyme or a dozen other herbs or spices that at the moment sounded like they might blend well. Create cold fusion."

"You mean you don't *remember*?"

"Are you kidding? Of course not! And I don't care. If it's possible, I'll taste whatever I'm cooking while I'm cooking it. If not, like if I'm spicing something raw, then I'll just play. Just have fun. And most of the time it works and some of the time it doesn't—and," he said, quickly turning to Janice with a raised warning finger, "I don't want to talk about any of my flavor disasters."

"Paprika on broiled strawberries," Janice whispered behind her hand to Karen.

"One strawberry! And it was a test."

"You see?" Janice said. "That's what I mean. His creativity in the kitchen is nothing more than simply being fearless."

"I could never cook like that," Karen said. "I'm the type who needs a recipe, something to follow."

"Then don't let all this talk of creativity in the kitchen scare you," Janice said. "Now you have my father's favorite cookbook, the one he followed to the letter for years, until he got brave enough to use the ideas he learned there to make dishes of his own. Believe me, he didn't turn into a hotshot experimenting cook overnight! So following a recipe is fine, because in the end, whether you cook with or without a recipe, the meals you start selecting will develop into a sort of routine."

"Call it the house menu," Fowler said to Janice.

"I like that," Janice said. "The house menu." Then she said to Karen, "You see, even though now he's always continually making something new, having fun, there's still this core group of meals that we always have on hand, meals that have become our comfort foods, that have been tailored to fit within the guidelines of the habits. Meals that you can easily make following a recipe."

"Exactly," Fowler said. "Whether you follow a recipe or not doesn't matter, because just like me, you're still going to end up with your own core group of meals."

Karen looked puzzled.

Fowler said, "The core group of meals are the meals you'll make over and over because they're the meals the family asks for. The family favorites."

"And a lot of them aren't even real cooking meals," Janice said. "Not meals that need a major production."

"That's right," Fowler said. "Many of *our* core meals are made on the spot, in just a few minutes, like all my breakfasts or my whole range of salads or my tuna specialties made with lemon juice and lowfat mayonnaise and Dijon mustard."

"He loves tuna packed in water," Janice said. "If he's in a hurry, he'll just open a can, drain it and turn it into tuna cracker sandwiches with a side dish of his precut veggies and dip. Then he'll get back to whatever he's doing in five minutes." She shook her head. "Another good example, though, of something he prepares on the spot, and one of my favorites, is his Pasta Primavera made with evaporated skim milk, cornstarch and Parmesan cheese."

"Cornstarch and just about any liquid makes a great gravy or sauce," Fowler said. "There's absolutely no need for fat. And that's a tip I got from one of my favorite Web sites. Don't forget that. There are plenty of excellent nutrition resources out there to help us—TV shows, books, Web sites— and we should be taking advantage of all of them."

Janice said, "It's because of resources like that that my father can have his lazy times where he doesn't do any cooking. Because now there are all those meals in the freezer and the ingredients for meals that can be made in just minutes in the fridge and cupboards."

"That's the amazing part," Karen said, flipping through the cookbook as she ate. "Not only have books like this taught you how to turn fat-filled meals that everyone loves into meals that are as low in fat as possible, but you've also developed your system of beating being lazy by being on top of things, by keeping your freezer filled with delicious, throw-in-the-microwave-or-oven meals, and your cupboards filled with the ingredients for meals that can be made in minutes. You are one step ahead of the curve. When Gary and I aren't eating garbage frozen meals or the junk that fills our cupboards, we're ordering in."

"That's what Janice is talking about," Fowler said. "Though certain foods—call them experimental foods or holiday foods—come and go, there's a core set of foods, of meals, eight, ten, twelve maybe, that every family eats over and over again—and enjoys just as much each time. The difference with us is that our core set of foods, our comfort foods, are built around the concepts of the eight habits."

"And life goes on seamlessly," Janice said. "The Power of One Good Habit goes to the core of our menu, takes over, and just disappears."

Fowler smiled. He finished his pepper, wiped his mouth on a napkin, took a deep swallow of water, and sat back. "We were supposed to be talking about the next habit," he said. He looked at Karen and her plate that was still mostly full, and added, "But before we do that, I want to know how you're doing with all that food. And even more importantly, I want to know if you're still starving."

# Twenty-Seven

Karen looked into Fowler's eyes. She had no answer to his question.

Once again Fowler asked, "Are you still starving?"

Karen dropped her eyes to the food on her plate. She'd tasted each of the items, but had eaten only about a third of the total amount, about as much food as Fowler had eaten. Left on Fowler's plate were just a few forkfuls of the Hearty Bean and Pasta Stew.

"The answer to the question isn't on the plate," Fowler said. "You're going to have to look somewhere else." He caught Janice's eye and raised one eyebrow.

Janice responded immediately. "If you're not still starving, if you can't say that, then are you at least still hungry? The way I was hungry?"

Karen frowned. She had her fork in her hand with a piece of turkey loaf speared through it. "This is really good food. I mean, *really* good."

Fowler laughed lightly. "That wasn't the question. The question was, are you still hungry? Is your stomach still telling you it needs food? You know, is it still growling? Still feeling sort of knotted? Is it still yelling its little stomach-head off demanding food?" He waited a moment, got no response, then said once more, "I'm not going to tell you that you have to stop eating. But just do this for me—put down your fork, take a good swallow of your water, and answer the question. Are you still hungry?"

Karen did as Fowler asked. She placed her fork back on her plate, took a swallow of her water, thought for a moment, and then said, "You know, the question *Are you hungry?* is something that people ask so often, I sort of forget it's a question. It's more of an invitation to eat. But once you start eating—once *I* start eating—there's never a point where I ask myself if I'm still hungry. Being not hungry is *not* the reason for me to stop eating. That's not when I say, 'Okay, I've had enough.' Being not hungry is not the trigger that gets me to put down my fork. Do you know what I mean?"

"I understand perfectly," Fowler said. "I was that way too. Sometimes I still am! Remember, I'm you. And being not hungry, having enough food in our stomachs so that it's stopped shouting for more, is not why we stop eating."

"You said that you're always starving," Janice pointed out. "Can you think about that statement again? Can you still say you're always starving?"

Karen smiled. "That, at least, I can answer. And the answer is no. I'm not always starving. I mean, even though I said it, and even meant it then, it's not true. How can anyone who eats regularly always be starving? Right now, I'm not starving. I'm not sure what I am. But I'm not starving. And with very little thought I can tell you there are times when I'm just the opposite of starving, when I'm stuffed."

"When you've swallowed the lead-filled beach ball," Janice said.

"What?"

"The lead-filled beach ball. At least, that's how my father

describes it." She looked at Fowler and smiled. "He has a name for everything, and that's what he calls it when we eat so much we can barely move."

"Barely walk or talk or breathe," Fowler said. "When you have to stumble to a couch and collapse onto it and sit there with your belt open and legs spread and lower jaw hanging, sucking back air while this lead-filled beach ball you just forced down your gullet crushes you. And then you wait, and moan, and wait, until your body begins to digest some of it, begins to give you some relief. It's completely ridiculous, but to differing degrees, that's what most of us call eating well. Satisfying our appetites. That's what I used to do." He laughed.

Karen didn't laugh with him. "You're describing *me*," she said. "I'll eat until I can't eat anymore. I don't even think about it. If it's there, I eat it. I eat until the plate's empty, no matter how much was on it—or until the baking dish is scraped clean—or until the bag of chips is gone—or until every container of the take-out food is picked through. I won't stop eating until there's nothing left to eat. And it has nothing to do with still being hungry. Of course I'm not still hungry; I'm *stuffed*! I've eaten the beach ball, and even then, if there's something else, some cookies or cake or ice cream or a piece of anything sweet left over from yesterday, I'll try to get that into my stomach too."

"I know what you're saying," Fowler said. "There was a time when food was an obsession for me. Stimulation. Adventure. Something to look forward to, even plan for. But not in the way I look forward to or plan for now. It was much bigger then. Wide-screen. Technicolor."

He pushed his chair slightly back from the table and crossed one leg over the other. "I used to think, Okay, tomorrow I'm going to buy that new book I've been wanting to read, and to make the reading of it better, more exciting, I'm going to get a double-size family pack of fried chicken and fries and the junk that comes with it, and read and eat for one, two, three hours, nonstop. And I would do just that!

Slowly but steadily stuff myself until I was ready to burst. And then I'd feel sick, sometimes literally—and sometimes just sick at heart about how I could have done that." He shrugged. "I ate that way for years. Doubling your weight takes that kind of effort."

"I do the same thing," Karen said in a small voice. "But I thought I was the only one." She reached for Gabe and stroked his hand. For now he was calm, content to just watch and listen.

Fowler shook his head. "You're not alone. You're the same as everyone out there who's lost control. We eat until we're stuffed, then watch TV, hit a commercial, maybe an ad for food, another cruise missile aimed into our homes, then eat some more. And on and on. But that behavior, using food as a crutch, as entertainment, as stimulation—eating until there's nothing left to eat, trying to satisfy ourselves and never really doing it—isn't caused by the enemy."

He smiled. "But that isn't to say that the enemy doesn't use it! We can feel how they use it with every commercial. Those advertisers lock onto us with their big guns. Competing with each other to see who can seduce us the quickest with the largest servings or the thickest steak or the most selections in their all-you-can-eat fat factories."

Janice said, "They know how our minds work. They're experts at that."

"They are!" Fowler agreed. "They know our weaknesses. And they zero in on them, using them to seduce us into their arms, their brightly colored, kid-friendly homes-away-from-home, where they batter us and our children over and over by offering every kind of artery-clogging, obesity-creating food they can make a buck on!" Fowler took a deep breath. "But the one thing the enemy doesn't do is stand over us with a gun and say, *Eat!*"

"Can I blame them anyway?" Karen asked, smiling sheepishly.

"You can blame anyone you want," Fowler said, "as long as you realize the answer to this particular problem is in here." He tapped his head. "You have to think it through. The key to the solution, just like the basic key to all the habits, is knowledge. Knowing what's behind your need to keep eating. Understanding what your body's telling you. Listening to it while you're eating."

Janice smiled at Karen. "Why don't we start again? The question we asked you was, 'Are you still hungry?' But before you answer it, I want you to talk to yourself. Think about it, and take your time. Then, if you decide that your feeling of being hungry is gone, and you still haven't stepped into lead-filled-beach-ball territory—I want you to stop eating." Then she quickly added, "But don't look for a feeling of being *satisfied*. That's not what I'm telling you to do. What I want is for you to look for a feeling of not needing to eat anymore. Not *needing* to eat, starting to get full. And if you have that feeling, then stop."

"Or take another bite," Fowler said. "But know that if you're not hungry anymore, if you've reached the point that Janice just described, of not feeling hungry, of starting to feel full, then know that that next bite is the one that'll cause your body to say to all its major parts, Hey, guys! Get ready! Because the boss is about to shove more food down her throat! Even though we already have plenty, more than enough to do our jobs, there's still more on the way! So everyone to your stations, because we're going to have to take that next bite and store it, just in case of famine. And for today we'll store it on her hips. And maybe tomorrow we'll pack it into a new chin."

"Stop eating," Janice urged.

"Take another bite," Fowler said. "Just one more. It's so good. Mmm-mmm. Food. Tasty food."

Karen laughed. She shook her head and picked up her fork and looked at the piece of turkey loaf still on it. "You little devil! You tempting little devil!"

"Habit Number Six," Fowler said. "Stop eating when you come to the point where you're not hungry anymore, when you're just beginning to feel full, and don't have even one more bite. No matter how much food is left on your plate, whether it's only a sliver of turkey loaf or still enough to feed an army, don't have even one more bite. And this is the hardest of the eight habits to follow. The one that for me, at the beginning, involved the greatest inner battle. But just like the other habits, it got easier and easier with each new device I put into place to tailor it, to make it work for me, for my personality. Work to the degree I wanted it to work at the moment. In the situation."

"He got creative with it," Janice said. "And he had to, because with this habit he's not fighting common sense, he's fighting genetics."

"I had to think it through," Fowler agreed. "Debate my genes. Use knowledge to fight instinct."

"What do you mean?" Karen asked.

Janice said, "The reason I said to stop eating when you feel *not* hungry, when you're just *starting to feel full*, and not when you feel satisfied, is because, genetically, we're programmed to eat everything in front of us. Genetically, and socially too, we're not going to be satisfied until all the food on our plate is gone. That's why it's so easy to get into lead-filled-beach-ball territory. It's part of our survival instinct. Eat all you can, in case of famine."

"When it comes to eating," Fowler said, "feeling satisfied and being not hungry are two completely different things. Think about it. If you've got tempting food in front of you, like now, your body is screaming, 'Eat it! We don't know when we'll get this stuff again. Eat it, because we won't be satisfied until it's all gone!'"

He took a good swallow of his water. "But your body isn't saying, 'Eat it because we're still starving.' That feeling of starvation is gone. And now you're trying to know if you have the feeling of even being just plain hungry. And *that's* what you've got to pick out. And you've got to do it while your body is screaming, Eat the stuff so we can store it for the next big famine!"

Janice smiled, but Karen wasn't smiling. She was staring at Fowler.

"One of the problems is that the food is still there," Fowler continued. "Still in front of you. That's the reason your body is still yelling. Because it can see it. Smell it. Still taste it on your taste buds. So your genetics, your instincts, all those parts, are continually yelling, Hey, good stuff! Eat! Eat! Keep on eating!"

Janice whispered to Karen, "Gabe's eyes are closing."

Karen turned to Gabe for a moment and stroked his cheek, but her focus was fully on Fowler.

Fowler said, "So you can see why, with this habit, with the concept of 'once I've got my hunger covered I won't eat another bite,' my creativity had to kick in. Big time! Beginning with a lot of talking to myself. And *that* was forced on me by my genetics. Genetics forced me to talk to my head. Talk to my instincts. Talk to my courage. And then use my brains."

Janice was nodding.

Karen asked, "What did you say to yourself?"

"The first thing I said is what I already told you. I asked myself, 'Where, exactly, do I want that next bite of food to go? Back to my belly? My thighs? To that roll I used to have under my chin?' It's got to go somewhere, so I thought of where, and that pitted those guys yelling for more food against my mirror."

"Did that work?"

He shrugged. "Sometimes." Karen laughed.

Fowler said, "But I also told myself that what I had sitting on my plate in front of me was only food. It may have been great food, even exceptional food, but in the end, it's still only food, and there'll always be more. Another meal. And another. And another. Forever and ever, until my last day. You see, what I was trying to do for my head was to put what was left on my plate into perspective. There's no shortage of food: we'll never see that. Not even of the great stuff. We're never going to have a famine, not in this country. So I tried to tell that to my genetics, say to them, 'Calm down, guys. Relax. Quit taking your work so seriously.'"

"Did that work?"

"Sometimes." This time it was Janice who laughed.

"Another device I used was to experiment with that last bite," Fowler said. "If I wasn't sure whether I'd reached the point of not being hungry, I'd take another bite and wash it down with a good swallow of water. Then I'd think about how I was feeling, ask myself again, 'Are you still hungry?' And if I still wasn't sure, I'd take another bite and another good swallow of water, and I'd keep doing that, quietly, working only with myself, with my head, until I was sure that my feeling of hunger was gone. And being sure—at the beginning, at least—used to come only when I could already feel that I'd pushed myself into lead-filled-beach-ball territory. Then, of course, I'd get mad at myself about those last bites, about which one of them wasn't necessary, and swear not to do it again. To be on top of it the next time."

"Did that work?"

"Sometimes," Fowler said again with a smile. "What began to happen after a while, though, after a lot of talking back and forth with my head, was that I began to know three things. First, I began to know what feeling not hungry felt like. It's a quiet, calm feeling, approaching feeling full, but still a good distance away from feeling stuffed. It's as though, if I could put it on a monitor like they have in hospitals, the line would be just slightly wavy. No big deal one way or the other. And I started to turn that feeling into one that said, I'm satisfied, because I'm not feeling hungry. So I can stop. No big deal. Just stop."

He put his elbows on the table. "The second thing I began to know, which I learned over time and from experience, was just how much to put onto my plate. And I began using that experience, preparing to stop even before I started to eat. I would fill my plate with the amount I knew, from experience, that I'd need to eat to not feel hungry, then bulk it up with salad to trick those guys downstairs into thinking that there was a ton of food on the plate and that the boss was going to eat it all. And I would. But we're talking about a game here. With my head. And salad. Because the stuffed feeling you get from extra salad is not lead-filled-beach-ball territory. But you *do* feel full."

"You also experimented with plate sizes," Janice said. "Using smaller and smaller plates, and making them fuller and fuller."

Fowler laughed. "That's right. I'd forgotten about that." To Karen he said, "When I first began to focus on this habit, I did whatever I could, whatever I had to, because I knew that my genetics weren't going to put up a fair fight."

Karen asked, "What was the third thing you learned?" She had pulled out Gabe's blanket and her notebook from the diaper bag. She covered Gabe, shielding his eyes from the overhead light, and was now taking notes while Fowler talked.

"The third thing I learned, again from experience, from really focusing on this habit, and on myself and this business of eating and stopping eating, was that though it seemed hard to stand up, leave the table, stop putting food into my mouth, if I did it—if I left the table and went on with whatever else I had to do, even putting the food and dishes away—that feeling of needing to eat more disappeared. In seconds! Because it's not a true feeling. I mean, I know I could still have pushed down a second helping of what I'd just eaten if I let myself. But that strong urge was gone. For then, at least. Until the next time I legitimately felt hungry."

Janice said, "Also remember, the message our stomach sends to our brains through our digestive enzymes and hormones, to tell us we're starting to feel full, the message we're trying to listen for—takes about fifteen minutes. So if you eat too quickly, if you stuff yourself within those first fifteen minutes, you'll have eaten yourself into beach-ball territory before you even realize it. It'll only hit you after you're finished eating. So what you want to do is eat slowly. Slow enough so you can listen to what your stomach has to say while you're in the process of filling it up. Slow enough so you have your stomach fighting *for* you, and not *against* you."

Karen nodded. She stopped writing. "So, basically what you're saying, is that you did whatever you had to, to either *keep* temptation away, or to *take* it away."

"That's exactly it!" Fowler said. "That's what became my most important life adjustment to this habit. I kept, and I keep, temptation away. I work at creating a situation where it's easy to say, 'That was good. I'm not hungry anymore. I know I can still shove a lot more food down, but I don't have it in front of me—so I won't.'"

He finished his glass of water with lemon. Putting the glass on the table, and staring into Karen's eyes, he said, "And after a while it became easy. Much easier than I could have imagined, because most of what we eat are foods we eat over and over again. Those comfort foods we talked about. So now, from experience, I just know how much is enough. And that's become the strongest tool I rely on. Now, using the knowledge of how much is enough, has become second nature. Using that knowledge has made this habit, like all the others, become an invisible part of my life. I just do it now. There's no more great debate, no diet mentality, no worrying about being perfect and never any guilt about being human."

"Tell her about your pizza," Janice said.

"The pizza's a perfect example because I love it. And I eat it often. But when I eat it, I'll only serve myself two slices. It started out being four, then three, but now it's only two, because now I know that two slices of the size pizza I make, along with a large salad, is all I need to be able to say, That's it, the hunger's gone, I'm approaching feeling full, but still not even close to feeling stuffed."

He grinned. "And I also know that the rest of the pizza is still close at hand. No one is going to steal it from the fridge. It can be eaten at the next snack, or the next meal, or the next day. Or made again and again. Or replaced with something else."

184

He held up a hand. "I know what you're going to ask next," he said. "And that's: 'Does this work when I eat out?' You bet it does! Because besides using everything I've already told you, when I eat out, I also use the pick-and-choose method."

"What's that?" Karen asked, her pen again poised to take notes.

"It's exactly what it sounds like. I pick and choose what I want to eat. For example, it can be either bread *or* dessert, but not both. Or eggs with toast *or* hash browns, but not eggs and toast *and* hash browns. You see, I limit what I eat by picking what I'm in the mood for most at the moment, and leaving out what doesn't tempt me as much. And I also do this," he said. He lifted his napkin, unfolded it and gently placed it over the remaining bites of food on his plate. "There," he said. "Out of sight, out of mind. And this works well here and when I eat out."

Janice nodded at Fowler, then pointed to the fruit bowl.

Fowler smiled. "And," he added, winking at Janice, "there's also this device." He reached for the fruit bowl and slid it closer.

"*I* thought of this one," Janice said.

Fowler picked a Granny Smith apple out of the bowl, tossed it into the air, caught it, and took a bite, then said, "Janice taught me to change the taste in my mouth. Take away the yummy taste of the stew or the pizza or whatever I'd been eating, by having a fruit—Mother Nature's own dessert."

Karen, looking impressed, nodded. She read back from her notes. "The key here, the same as with the other habits, is to think ahead. Work with yourself until you know the right amount of food for you, and then make sure you have only that amount. Then walk away, knowing there's always the next snack or meal." She pressed her lips to a determined line, pushed the platter of food to the center of the table and reached for an orange. And smiled at Fowler.

"Exactly."

Janice looked at Fowler. "It was after learning this habit—to stop eating when you're no longer hungry and not take another bite—after you figured out the way to do that and make it a part of your life, that the Power of One Good Habit really took over. It was at this point that you stopped working at it and simply let it sweep you away."

"I remember that," Fowler said. "I hit a kind of critical mass. But it was really a culmination of the habits I knew up to then." To Karen he said, "I was already letting the excitement of any result I got from the habits push me forward. But by this habit, by the time I'd tailored this one so completely into my life that it disappeared, the Power of One Good Habit became . . . overwhelming."

Karen said, "I've just barely begun applying any of what I know so far, but I've also begun to see results. And I'm also beginning to *feel* something."

"That's exactly what I want," Fowler said. "But I don't want you to rush it. Don't push the habits. Let the habits push you. Take one tiny step, only one, then look around, see what you see, feel what you feel, know that that single step is a great success in itself. And then, when you're ready, take another step, and then another, and never let yourself fall into the diet-mentality trap. Never let any of it make you feel guilty or anxious or worried. Never."

"I'm ready for that now," Karen said. "What I'm feeling now is excitement. An expectation of something good about to happen." She paused for a moment and smiled. "And I'm planning on making a lot of that happen tomorrow night."

"You sound as though you're about to fly off on your honeymoon," Janice said.

"I do, don't I?" Karen laughed. "It's because that's what I'm feeling. That kind of excitement. And Gary doesn't know anything about it. I have the whole evening planned as a surprise. A fantasy evening for the two of us. One that includes the Power of One Good Habit."

# Twenty-Eight

"There. That's finished," Karen said, looking around the room with a sense of satisfaction. She walked over to Gabe's playpen, lifted him up and gave him a hug.

She'd begun her preparations first thing that morning, the moment Gary left for work: a room-by-room, corner-by-corner scrubbing. Now the townhouse was immaculate—and she knew she was one step closer to her goal of a total change. A change in herself and a change in her marriage.

She had been experimenting with the first four habits all week, testing how far she wanted to take them, and could already feel them becoming second nature. And starting today she had begun incorporating the two she learned yesterday.

Her excitement was growing, and she let that push her forward.

For breakfast she'd used only one egg yolk in her three-egg omelet, and alongside it had had an orange and lowfat cream cheese on whole-grain bread. For lunch her plate was full because she'd used Fowler's trick of serving herself on a smaller-than-usual plate. She had also begun to eat more slowly, taking the time to really appreciate the broiled orange roughy to which she had treated herself, along with a left-over sweet potato and a salad on the side.

Hugging Gabe once more, she thought, *Whether you know it or not, Gary, things are going to get better.*

He hadn't kissed her before he left for work; he hadn't done that since the first year of their marriage. But he had looked at her, given her what she thought was something close to a smile—an indication, at least, that the transformation he'd begun to see in her was starting to have an effect on him.

And that look, no matter how small and quick, had had an effect on *her.* Karen had wanted to run after Gary when he closed the door, reach him before he got to the car, tell him she knew it was going to work, that their marriage was going be good again, fresh and vibrant and loving and caring, the way it had been at the beginning. And that she was going to lose the weight—especially that, lose all the weight the enemy had seduced her into gaining; become finally, and this time permanently, the woman he'd married. And do it too because *she* wanted it, not just him.

She'd thought about this too, carefully, and knew that though the result was the same, that specific intention, her strong new mindset, changed everything.

But she hadn't run after him, because she knew words were too easy to say, and that she'd said them too often in the past. Knew too that those easy words usually produced a sarcastic, cutting response. This time, she decided, she was going to save her words—and *show* him, and herself, instead.

She carried Gabe into the kitchen, belted him into the high chair and gave him his colored rings to play with. The radio was on and she began to hum along with it, thinking, *Time to begin, to create my own Power of One Good Habit restau-*

*rant, to break down the habits into a form I can accept. Tailor them, the way Fowler taught me, to fit Gary's life and mine.*

"Choose foods that are as low in fat as possible," she'd written in her journal, "and then, for my health and Gary's, add back small amounts of good fat." *Simple enough,* she thought, knowing she was now on a hunt for fat.

She had to accommodate Gary. That was important. And herself, too. It was important to be aware of their comfort level. She would begin slowly, the way Fowler had begun, let her involvement in the habits build of its own momentum, be result-driven and not forced. This was not a diet. It required courage and thought and planning and choices—but no pain or sacrifice or any part of a diet mentality.

And since Gary left the food shopping and cooking—and virtually the kitchen itself—to her, the process of defatting, of creating her Power of One Good Habit haven, was hers alone. She was particularly glad about that.

She began with the obvious, replacing the butter and margarine with two pump sprayers for oil, one with olive oil, with its particular rich flavor, and the other with canola oil for its milder taste. In her journal she wrote: "Unless it's broiled, boiled, steamed or cooked on the outdoor grill, it'll be prepared with the least amount of fat possible!"

It was a good start, she knew, one that on its own would produce results. But she'd gone even further, replacing all the dairy products she used with similar items—but only those marked as being lowfat.

She realized, however, that though these initial steps were very positive, they were still the easy part of the battle to find and eliminate fat, just the scratching of the surface. The real battle was in the cooking itself, in her choice of foods and in the preparation. And in the ever-important adding back of good fats. But just like Fowler, she knew she could do it. She would use her new cookbook, along with common sense and creativity, to incrementally—and continuously, for the rest of her life—gain health for herself and her family.

"Okay," Karen said out loud. "What's next?"

She went to the refrigerator, opened the door and stared. Then she took out the mayonnaise. "I love you," she said, holding up the jar. "We've been late-night buddies for a very long time." But she knew there was a perfectly acceptable lowfat version of the mayo, and from now on, that was the only version she'd allow in her kitchen. She knew, too, that late-night snacking was also now off her list. If she needed something to quell her hunger before sleep, she'd have a piece of fruit or a few peanuts or almonds, and that way also add back the good fats Fowler had talked about.

She tossed the jar of mayonnaise into the garbage, then opened the door to the freezer. The package of toaster pastries went without a thought. Then she reached for the ice cream, but quickly pulled back her hand. In a conspiratorial whisper, she said to the frozen bucket, "You can stay there for now, but you'd better keep your nose clean, mister, because you are definitely on probation!"

She laughed, closed the freezer door and reached for her glass of water with lemon. She'd emptied a quart-size pitcher already today, and though she wasn't counting glasses, she was aware of her need to drink.

She'd weighed herself this morning, even though Fowler had told her not to do that more than once a week, even once a month. She understood his explanation. There could be daily weight fluctuations that had nothing to do with gaining or losing fat, and because of this, weighing herself too often left her open to a disappointing result that wasn't even true. "Wait until you hit your maintenance level like me," he'd said. "Then you can weigh yourself every day. That way you'll get an early alert to any slip-up and make sure it won't become a problem. And you can also keep reminding yourself of your success, and of your daily goal."

But she'd weighed herself anyway and was thrilled to see the scale had dropped another half pound. It was amazing, she thought, knowing she hadn't even put a fraction of what she was planning into effect. All she had done so far was focus on drinking water, on using mostly egg whites with hardly any yolks, and on eating breakfast first thing in the morning, replacing her doughnut with whole-wheat toast and lowfat cream cheese. She might have been satisfied with just that. Losing three pounds in one week with virtually no effort was just about miraculous.

But that loss of three pounds was now pushing her. Fowler was right. Results produced excitement, and excitement created an urge to achieve even greater results. And this urge was becoming the push for her to find even more ways to apply the six habits she'd learned so far.

Yesterday, as she was leaving Fowler's house, she had asked him to tell her what the last two habits were, but he said he wanted to wait until she had more time. "Work with what you already have," he said. "The last two are beauties. You're going to love them both. And I don't want to just hand them to you. I want to gift-wrap them first, present them as the prizes they are." He laughed at her curiosity, with Janice joining in.

Fowler had also talked about the importance of exercise, saying, "We have to always keep in mind our need to move. Just move. Whether it's in the garden or walking to the store from the far side of the parking lot or taking the stairs instead of the elevator. We have to move, and grab any chance we can to do it."

Well, she was going to do that too, Karen thought. Grab any chance to move. And she had done that this morning while cleaning the townhouse, and then again when she walked to the store with Gabe in his stroller to buy what she needed for tonight's meal. The old Karen would have automatically taken the car.

Tonight's meal! This was going to be the first complete as-low-in-fat-as-possible meal for her and Gary. It would be as-low-in-sugar-as-possible too. And no part of it would use processed or chemically enhanced ingredients. For her, it would also be a meal where she was going to serve herself only the amount she thought would take away her hunger—

that, and a hefty salad with lowfat dressing. And if she felt she was approaching being full before she'd eaten everything on the plate, she'd stop eating; stop then, at that moment, and not have even one more bite.

She had already done it this morning for breakfast. And then again for lunch. She had listened to her stomach, thinking it through, the way Fowler had taught her. And for both meals she'd carried the plate to the sink and emptied the last few bites without eating them because she had had enough. Fowler was right. It was hard! It took a conscious effort. But once she'd done it, the moment she'd done it, the thought of that food was gone. Just gone. And she was on to other things. It was at that moment that she knew for certain that from this point on, life was going to be different!

She glanced at the clock. Although there was still plenty of time, she wanted to begin preparing the meal early, so she could allow herself room to experiment. "Courage and creativity," she said aloud. "Those are my defenses. And the habits are my weapons."

Using Fowler's worn cookbook as a guide, she had thought out the menu carefully. And she had thought out the evening, as well.

What Karen was hoping for tonight was simply for Gary to realize she was there. That she existed. That would be a positive first step. She envisioned them eating the meal together in the dining room, with Gabe in his high chair between them. The stereo would be playing softly and the television would be off. She was going to use the good dishes, light the fancy candles. She wanted to create a warm atmosphere. Most of all, though, what she wanted was to talk.

Just talk.

About anything.

It had been so long since Gary had told her how his day had gone, who'd done what or said what. It had been so long since he'd sighed and leaned back in his chair with his hands crossed behind his head and told her one of the dreams he had for their future—the cottage in the country, time to go fishing, time to be together.

She wanted to see him smile, hear him laugh, watch him once again become the man she had married. The man with the quick sense of humor, with shoulders she could lean on. The man who was caring with her, conscious of her needs. The man with whom she had fallen in love.

"We can do it, Gary," she whispered. "*I* can do it. I know I can. With Fowler's help, with the Power of One Good Habit, it'll change. You'll see."

She kissed Gabe on the forehead, rattled his rings, offered him a teething biscuit, then picked it up off the floor when he decided he wasn't hungry.

The menu Karen had planned with the recipes from her new book was quick and easy. *Keep it simple,* she'd told herself. *This meal is going to become our first new core meal, a healthy core meal to replace any of the meals we live on now, any one of those high-fat mistakes, the burgers and French fries, or fried chicken with gravy, or take-out pizza or Chinese. This meal is going to become a new staple, a new comfort food.*

She nodded determinedly. While shopping today she'd kept in mind what Janice had said. "The less junk food we buy, the less they'll make. The more healthy foods we buy, the more they'll make. Changing our culture has to begin with knowledge—acted-on knowledge, because only then can we, the people, make a change—by voting with our dollars."

Today, Karen knew, she had done her part.

She took six skinless chicken breasts from the refrigerator, removed all the visible fat and cleaned them.

Gary, she knew, could eat two. She would eat one, and then see. And the other three would go into her energy bank. She smiled. She was starting an energy account. She would make her first deposit in the freezer tonight and begin to build up her capital there, while compiling all the items she wanted to have on hand in the refrigerator and cupboards for those simple nutritious meals she could make in just minutes. From now on, she would be prepared! She wouldn't let the excuse of fatigue interfere with her progress. No excuse was going to break her stride!

*I'm going to let the habits work for me,* she thought. *I'm going to let the excitement they're creating push me into taking each of them to the greatest degree my comfort level allows—without falling into the diet-mentality trap. I'm going to let their force build until it becomes so ingrained in my life that it becomes . . . invisible.*

*And it'll happen! It will! The same way it did for Fowler. And it'll work for Gary too, even if he won't know what's happening until he begins to see his own results.* She smiled, picturing Gary's face when she eventually told him why they were both losing weight and gaining health, knowing that something as positive as the new habits couldn't possibly get a negative reaction, not even from Gary. What had Fowler said? *It's hard to argue about something that feels good.* Well, losing weight and gaining health were certainly going to feel good!

"Seamlessly," she whispered. *That's how it works for Fowler and Janice, and that's how it's going to work for us. There's no apparent difference in the way they live their lives now and the way they lived their lives before incorporating the eight habits. No apparent difference—except that Fowler lost enough weight to build his own twin!*

*Okay,* she thought, placing the cleaned chicken breasts aside. *Get creative, get the juices flowing. I'm serving two very important guests tonight, VIPs of the highest order—my husband and me!*

# Twenty-Nine

Karen's first thought was to make the crunchy potato wedges Fowler loved. She found that recipe in her new book, knowing it would be a perfect replacement for the fat-filled French fries Gary could eat seven nights a week. But then she decided to try something different. She smiled, knowing Fowler would be proud of her courage and creativity.

One of Gary's favorite dishes, she knew, was scalloped potatoes. For him it was a comfort food from years ago, a dish his grandmother used to make for him and his brother. *The only thing is, first his grandmother, then his mother and me, used butter and fat-filled cheddar cheese and whole milk to prepare it.* "That's just not acceptable anymore," she said aloud. "Think, girl. You can do this."

She began by peeling, then thinly slicing, the potatoes and a couple of onions. Then, instead of buttering her baking dish the way she normally would, she used the pump oil sprayer to lightly cover it with canola oil, thinking, *Replace the bad fat with small amounts of the good.*

Next she sautéed flour spiced with salt and pepper in a small amount of oil, then to this added skim milk that only yesterday would have been fat-laden whole. She had decided to go down the milk fat scale quickly after Janice figured out for her that simply switching from whole to skim for the glass or so she drank every day, plus the milk in her cereal, could mean the loss of twelve or more pounds in a year.

She stirred the flour-and-milk mixture until it began to bubble lightly, then set it aside. Next she layered about a third of the potatoes into the baking dish, covered this with a few slices of the onion, then topped it off with a nice handful of lowfat grated cheddar cheese.

"Looking good," she said, as she repeated the process, adding a second layer of potatoes to the dish. Once this was done, she poured in the flour-and-milk mixture so that it covered the potatoes, and then finished the dish by sprinkling more lowfat cheddar over it, and topping the cheddar with a Fowler-like flourish of dried parsley.

"You," she said aloud to herself, carrying the baking dish to the oven, "are one creative genius!" Then she laughed, knowing the process of turning a fat-filled meal into one that had as little fat as possible was so simple that even Gabe, if he could read, if he could stand, would have been able to do it. *Anyone could do it,* she thought—if they knew the words to the first habit. *As low in fat as possible, then where you can, add back small amounts of good fat for your health. Change the butter to canola oil from the pump sprayer. Whole milk to skim. Regular cheese to lowfat.* All she had to do was follow Fowler's favorite saying: "knowledge is power, and we have choices." *It's a matter of choices, of preparing in advance to have those items on hand, of creating a lowfat haven.* "Thank you, Fowler," she said, before turning once again to the chicken.

The dish she was about to make was Chicken Marsala, another of Fowler's standards, from his favorite cookbook.

She cut an onion into wedges, chopped two cloves of garlic, drained a can of mushrooms, then sautéed these ingredients in one tablespoon of olive oil for a few minutes before adding the cleaned skinless chicken breasts to the frying pan.

*A snap*, she thought.

Then came the chicken broth, cornstarch and spices, and finally, one-third of a cup of Marsala wine.

"Go for it, girl!" she said happily while the Chicken Marsala simmered.

The radio was playing. Her hips were swaying. She played a funky little beat with her wooden spoon against the side of the sauté pan.

Then she thought, *veggies*, not needing to refer to her notes to remember that Fowler had talked about a reasonable portion of as-low-in-fat-as-possible protein, alongside a potato, pasta or rice, and then a deeply colored vegetable or two, plus the salad. Janice had called this the true key to health through nutrition. A protein at every meal and snack to keep blood sugar levels even, and a variety of foods for all the vitamins and minerals and cancer-fighting antioxidants they provided.

The natural order of our meals, Fowler had added. Well-rounded, well-balanced, tasty and satisfying—the exact opposite of gimmicky fad diets designed to twist our heads into a knot and our willpower into pretzels.

Karen went to the freezer, took out a package of frozen green beans and got them steaming. Then she did the same to a package of baby carrots. Both packages were free of oil, butter or sauce. Then she opened a bag of fresh salad, poured it into a bowl, added a handful of cherry tomatoes and cucumber slices and a dash of lowfat dressing, and said aloud, "You've done it! One unbelievable Power of One Good Habit meal—in lickety-split time!"

She suddenly felt like celebrating, then realized, *It's not the effort, that's not the reason to celebrate. Because there was no effort. None beyond what I would usually have spent to make any meal. It's the fact that this meal will add to our health. That this meal, which is actually two meals, because I made enough to bank both the chicken and the potatoes in the freezer, will cause us to lose weight.*

"We have to eat to lose weight," she said, repeating what Fowler had told her. *You were right, Fowler. It's the knowledge that's powerful, because that knowledge gives us the power of choice. And those simple choices will change my life and turn me into the woman I want to be!*

*And I can hardly wait!*

When the chicken was ready, she put it into a baking dish to be kept warm in the oven alongside the scalloped potatoes and beans and baby carrots that she had spiced and tossed in a quick spray of olive oil. Then she prepared the dining room table with the good dishes and two candles, and changed the music from the radio to a CD.

By the time she heard Gary open the front door, she had changed, put on makeup and a hint of perfume, had just finished changing Gabe and was now placing him into his high chair at the dining room table.

Gary first walked into the kitchen, then the dining room.

Karen, in a soft, hopeful voice, said, "Hi."

"What's going on?" Gary wanted to know.

"Nothing's going on," Karen said. "I just thought we'd do something different tonight."

Gary looked at the table, at the setting, the candles, then at Karen. He appeared bewildered. Then his expression changed to something closer to amusement. Karen smiled in response.

But Gary's amusement lasted only seconds. He said, "You're ridiculous, and I won't be a part of it." And with that he turned, left the room and in a moment slammed the front door to the townhouse. Even from the dining room, Karen could hear his tires screeching as he spun out of the driveway.

For one long minute, then two, then five, Karen did not move. Her expression stayed blank. Then she swallowed hard and said to Gabe, "It's all right. It's just the first try. It took

198

time for it to get bad, and it'll take a bit of time for it to get good again. But it will. You'll see, it will."

She stood up, walked to the kitchen, took out the pan of scalloped potatoes and the one filled with the Chicken Marsala and the third with the green beans and baby carrots, and very calmly scraped all three pans into the garbage. Then she went to the drawer, found a spoon, went to the freezer, took out the ice cream and walked back to the dining room.

—

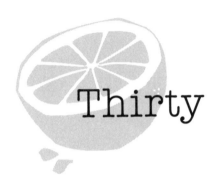

# Thirty

Karen stood on Fowler's back porch, holding Gabe in her arms. She could hear Fowler's voice, his words muffled, coming from somewhere inside the house. Then she heard Janice saying clearly, "I can't!"

For a moment Karen hesitated, unsure whether to stay or return home. Then she forced herself to knock. Courage's welcoming bark brought an agitated Fowler to the door.

It had been ten days since she had last been here. Ten days since she had declared herself ready to be her own person, able to choose her own friends, decide whether or not the Power of One Good Habit was for her. Ten days since she'd vowed to fight for her health and her marriage.

And she had fought.

And Gary had fought back, first by ridiculing her efforts and her weight, then by shutting her out of his life through a silent treatment so complete it virtually paralyzed her, left her able to manage only a couple of short, tear-filled calls to Janice. Then none at all.

Last night Gary had come home at three in the morning and told her to get out of his bed, saying that he wouldn't sleep with her anymore. "From now on, you can sleep on the couch!"

After Gary left for work, Karen had taken the shortcut through the woods to Fowler and Janice's house. She was struggling through another morning-after-the-fight daze. But this time, she knew, things were different. This time she had no fight left in her. She was tired: emotionally battered and drained. And this time, too, she weighed more than when she'd last been here. *I'm numb*, she thought. *Resigned to whatever Gary wants to throw at me. I've gone beyond hopelessness. There's nothing left. No courage. None.*

On top of it all, this morning, for the first time, Karen found the mood tense at Janice and Fowler's.

Fowler ushered her in, then slipped behind the counter as Karen took a seat next to Janice. Though the baby seat was on the table she decided to keep Gabe in her lap. "What can I get you for breakfast?" Fowler asked. He wore a troubled expression and there were no pleasantries from him for either of the two women.

At the table, Janice had an untouched cup of tea in front of her and nothing else. No books, no papers, no magazines. Even the newspaper she usually read lay unopened.

Karen sighed uneasily, knowing something was wrong. *Coming here was a mistake,* she thought. *They have their own problems today. No, I'm not going to eat here, not going to stay, not going to learn the rest of the habits. All I'm going to do is go back home and rewind the tape of my marriage, then play it over and over over . . .* She cleared her throat and said to Fowler. "No thank you. Nothing for me. Not today. I won't be having breakfast today."

Janice looked at her. "Breakfast is one of the habits."

Karen shook her head. "No. I have no habits. Not anymore."

Fowler stared at her, then stepped past the counter to the table but didn't take his seat.

Karen dropped her eyes, "I'm sorry. I know you don't want to hear this. But there are no habits for me. Not for me."

"If there are no habits," Janice asked, "then what is there?"

Fowler crossed his arms over his chest. His expression was grim. Suddenly he clapped his hands once, and said forcefully, "What there is, is breakfast out! At someone else's restaurant. With someone else's food. On my tab. And we're going now!"

Janice turned her head to Fowler and looked at him as though he'd just spoken in a strange language.

"Now!" Fowler said. "I mean it. The day is young and I feel great and I want to get going." He gazed steadily into Janice's eyes.

Janice began to say, "I'll wait for you—"

"You're not waiting anywhere," Fowler interrupted. "I said *we're* going out. The four of us. And you have five minutes to get ready or I'm going to put on my khaki shorts with my cowboy boots and miner's lamp. And if you think one unusually shaped woman with a beautiful smile, one slightly overweight woman who's lost track of her habits and one perfect little boy are a sight, you're going to have to live with that, too." He didn't laugh. Neither did Janice or Karen.

Janice said, again, "I can't."

"You can!" Fowler said. He turned to Karen. "Other than trips to the hospital, Janice has never left this house. Not once in twenty-six years. I'm to blame for some of that time. But not all of it."

Janice whispered, "I can't. I'm sorry. I can't face other people." She turned to Karen and began to say, "I'm a freak—"

"No!" Karen cried, sitting upright as though she'd been jolted with an electric shock. *That's the word Gary used once to describe me!*

202

"It's the truth," Janice said. "You don't see it anymore. But I *am* a freak. Nothing but a—"

"Stop saying that!" Karen shouted, suddenly breaking into tears, unable to hear Janice describe herself this way. She reached for Janice's hand and held it tightly. Courage stood, ready to defend his friend..

Fowler's jaws were tightly clamped. In a strong serious tone, he said, "Okay. I want both of you to listen very carefully to what I'm going to say . . . We've done a lot of talking during the past few weeks, and we covered a lot of topics. We talked about courage and creativity. About the Power of One Good Habit. About choices. But what we haven't talked about are walls: getting through the walls we're all inevitably going to find in our way. The walls blocking our chosen path, holding us back."

Tears were running down Karen's cheeks. "How do we get through those walls?" she asked. "What's the answer?"

"The only way to get through any wall," Fowler said, "is to do it. Confront the wall. Do what needs to be done. And take it down."

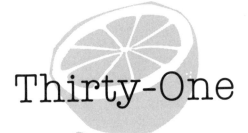

# Thirty-One

Karen got into the back seat with Gabe, while Fowler
helped Janice into the front. He folded Janice's
portable wheelchair and placed it in the car's trunk.
Courage, his nose pressed against the living room window,
barked anxiously.

Karen's eyes were still moist.

Janice wept quietly. She'd first said no, then yes, then no
again, then changed her mind one last time to a final yes—
and stuck to it. "But I'm afraid," she whispered then, "more
afraid than I've ever been in my life."

Fowler, putting the car into drive, said, "Boy, talk about
your happy outings!"

Fowler waited in front of Karen's townhouse while Karen
got Gabe's car seat from her own car and her tote bag of baby
supplies. She snapped the seat into the back seat of Fowler's
and adjusted Gabe securely. Although there was no one
around, Janice sat hunched down in the front seat.

Fifteen minutes later, Fowler turned into the parking lot of the Family Style restaurant. He pulled into the handicapped parking spot. No one said anything.

Fowler got the wheelchair from the trunk and lifted Janice from the car to the chair, covering her lap and legs with a blanket. Only now did Janice say to Karen, "Please stay close to me."

"I'm right here," Karen answered her. "I'll be beside you the whole time." She picked Gabe up and balanced him on her right hip, then slung the diaper bag over her left shoulder.

Fowler guided Janice's wheelchair to the access ramp and up and through the automatic doors, where the hostess met them. "Hello," she said cheerfully. "Will that be four?" Then she looked at Janice and her smile died. She snapped her eyes away, looked back again, then focused wide-eyed on Fowler's hard expression.

It was Karen who said, "Yes, four, and we'll need a high chair for the baby, please."

Janice's eyes remained lowered.

The hostess, a pretty woman in her twenties, replied, "Oh, yes. Right away." She showed them to a corner table where she cleared a place for the wheelchair while studiously avoiding another glance at Janice.

Fowler moved Janice to the table. The hostess left, then quickly returned with the high chair and three menus. She placed the menus on the table, asking, "Coffees all around?"

"Please," Fowler said.

"Perfect," the hostess replied. "Your server will be with you in just a few minutes. Enjoy your meal."

"Thank you," Fowler answered.

Karen strapped Gabe into the high chair, and then sat down adjacent to Janice. Fowler was sitting across from Karen.

Janice's eyes were still cast low. She reached for her menu but did not open it. Instead she touched Karen's arm and in a whisper said to her, "Is anyone looking?"

Karen turned toward the other customers in the restaurant.

There were eyes on Janice, most discreetly, a few less so. For a moment Karen too dropped her head, only to look up into Fowler's tense expression.

Fowler said, curtly, "She asked you a question and I think she deserves an answer."

Karen turned to Janice. "Yes," she said, "some people are looking." She put her hand on Janice's shoulder.

Janice was trembling. She lowered her head even further.

A woman server stepped up to the table with three coffees and placed them, saying, "Good morning! How's everyone doing?"

Karen mumbled, "Fine." Fowler nodded his head. The server asked, "You all ready to order yet?" Karen could tell she had been briefed by the hostess about Janice, because she didn't even blink at Janice's appearance. Janice kept her head low.

"No," Karen answered. "We'll need a few more minutes."

"Sure thing," the server said. "Take all the time you need."

The moment she left, Janice said, head still bowed. "I have to leave."

Fowler was looking at her. He remained silent.

Karen put her hand on Janice's arm. "But we're already here," she said gently. "The hardest part is over. You took the first step, you found the courage to do that. For the first time in your life, you left your house to go someplace other than the hospital, knowing what to expect. And now you're here, at your wall." She paused for a moment, then, squeezing Janice's arm, said, "Confront it, Janice. Do what your father said. Face it. Take down your wall."

Again Karen looked at Fowler. He was nodding at Janice, urging her to take Karen's advice. Suddenly Karen realized that what she had just done for Janice was describe what she herself needed to do. *In exactly the same way that being overweight controls my life,* she thought, *Janice's fear controls hers.*

*And the process to overcoming both is the same. Find the courage, go with the knowledge, take that first step—and then confront any wall that gets in the way.*

Janice, her head still bowed, voice low and filled with pain, said, "You don't know what it feels like. You can't."

"Then tell us," Fowler said. "You're right: we don't know how it feels. You have to tell us."

"It feels like I'm on display," Janice replied, her voice breaking now. "Like I'm a sideshow—"

"Don't say that!" Karen begged, not wanting Janice to use the word *freak* again. "Please don't say that."

"No," Fowler said. "Not that. We already know that, and we understand. And you're right. To a certain extent you *are* on display, at least for a little while. Janice, you look different from the rest of us. You have a disability most people have never before seen. And people are curious. That's just human nature. We know all that. We came in here knowing that, knowing what to expect. And now you've hit a difficult moment. You're at your wall. And I want to know what *that* feels like. That part that only *you* can feel."

Janice lifted her head slightly and looked at Fowler. "What do you mean?"

"I mean, what does it feel like to be at your wall? What does it feel like to be in the process, right now, as we speak, of breaking through your wall? I want to know what you're feeling now, at this exact moment." His voice had begun to rise. When the server walked up, he quickly waved her off, saying, "Sorry, we still need a few more minutes."

Janice was still staring at Fowler. It took her a moment before she said, speaking very slowly, "It feels as though I'm being eaten alive. As though all of my muscles are screaming, just screaming with pain. As though I'm forcing myself through a vat of thick, heavy acid. Burning acid. This process is slow, and painful, and every ounce of my being is crying out to not be here. I don't want to be here. I don't want the pain. I want to go home." She closed her eyes, let her tears fall. Then she opened her eyes abruptly and said, her voice too beginning to rise, "But I have no choice, do I? I can't just leave on my own. I'm here because I'm being forced to be here!"

For a moment Fowler said nothing. Then he reached across the table and took his daughter's hand. "You do have a choice," he said evenly, staring directly into Janice's eyes. "Say it again. Tell me once more that you want to leave. Once more. And I'll take you home. Take you out of this . . . process. This effort. Take you back to what you know, to where you can draw the curtains again and hide. Say it one more time—I want to leave."

Janice stared at her father.

"Say it now!" Fowler said.

Karen, thrusting out a suddenly clenched fist, said to him, "Don't you—!"

But Fowler cut her off. "You stay out of this! What do you know about what's happening here? There's no one, no one in this room, who has half the courage Janice has. No one! Only she doesn't know it. Not yet. She doesn't know that for twenty-six years I've looked to her to find my strength. That I've looked to her to get the strength I needed to be able to do the little I've done with my life!"

"I'll stay," Janice said suddenly.

Fowler turned to her. "Are you sure?"

"Yes. I don't want to go back. I'll go through the pain. I'll get through it. I don't want to go back. It's time to stop hiding." She gazed at her father.

Karen's eyes filled with tears.

Fowler said to Janice, "I love you."

"I know."

"I'm sorry."

"I'm not," Janice said. "I'm glad it happened." She lifted her head a little higher, turned it slightly toward Karen and said, "Thank you."

Karen nodded. Then she looked at Fowler and, after a long pause, said, "Everyone has walls, don't they? Walls of some kind?"

"Yes. Everyone has walls. In that way, we're all alike. The only difference is in how we handle our walls when we get to them."

Again, for a long moment, no one spoke. Karen knew that Fowler and Janice, like her, were taking in the enormity of what had just happened. Finally Karen said to Fowler, "An hour ago I told you I had no more habits. I had come up to my wall and let it stop me. But now—now I want my habits back. I'm ready to break through my wall."

She reached again for Janice's hand.

—〜—

# Thirty-Two

"Then take your habits back," Fowler said to Karen.

"Just like that?" Karen asked. Gabe began banging on the highchair table and she reached into her tote bag and took out his rings. He grabbed for them excitedly. Karen took a sip of her coffee.

"Yes. Just like that," Fowler said to Karen, also reaching for his coffee. "They're yours to take. They're a part of you now. And a part of the process of owning the Power of One Good Habit is using it, and walking away from it, and going back again, as many times as you need to."

"Is that what happened to you?"

"That's what's *still* happening to me! Karen, there's no end to walls, to obstacles, to difficult situations. We do our best, and sometimes our best isn't good enough, and we fall back on old ways. And then, when we can, we pick ourselves up and crash through the wall that jumped into our path, and move on. Knowing other walls will come up. Walls that we'll handle as we get to them." Fowler shook his head. "Karen, this is real life not playtime. Diets are playtime. You go to the playground, play the diet, struggle under the diet mentality, then go home—go back to real life. The Power of One Good Habit *is* real life. And real life isn't always pretty. We fall down and scrape our knees. Then get back up and move on. And our habits move on with us—continue to move on—for the rest of our lives." He met Janice's eyes and smiled at her.

"So I can try again?" Karen said.

"No," Fowler said quickly, turning back to Karen. "You can *do* it again."

Karen stared at him, then took a deep breath and, in a determined voice, said, "Then the habits are mine again. I reclaim them!"

"Good. That's what I wanted to hear."

"All six of them."

The server came up to the table. "You folks ready yet?" she asked. The three menus had still not been opened. For the moment, food did not seem to be on anyone's mind. Fowler said to her, "I think we'll just stick with our coffees for a little while, just until we finish our meeting."

"No problem," the server said. "Take all the time you need. I'll be back soon to refill your coffees."

When she walked off, Fowler said to Karen, "Do you remember that I told you the last two habits were gifts?"

"I do! And I've wanted to know what you meant by that ever since you said it! How could something you're supposed to do when it comes to eating be considered a *gift*?"

"They *are* gifts. Believe me." Fowler glanced at Janice again. Her head was fully raised now and she was slowly, cautiously looking around the room. He pressed his fingers around hers and whispered, "Are you okay?"

"Yes," she answered. "It's getting better."

Fowler squeezed her hand once more. Then he leaned back in his seat with his coffee cup in hand, and said to Karen, "Okay, let me ask you something: what's the best thing about eating?" He took a sip of his coffee, saying to Janice, "It's good. Fresh. Try it." Janice reached for her cup.

"The best thing about eating," Karen said to Fowler, "is just . . . eating!"

"That's right," Fowler said.

"It is?"

"Of course it is! The best thing about eating is eating. I love to eat. You love to eat. *Everyone* loves to eat. And the reason the seventh habit is a gift is because it says just that: Eat often."

"Eat often? How can that be?"

Fowler smiled. "The human body wasn't designed to survive on just three meals a day. That's a rule society came up with. And it's a rule all of us can ignore. What you really want to do is eat five or six times a day. Every two or two and a half or three hours. Whatever's convenient. However, the habit can be tailored to suit your needs at the time."

"Eat five or six times a day?"

"That's right. Remember when we invited you for lunch and you said you were starving? And Janice and I said we were hungry, but not starving? Well, that's one of the problems with eating only three times a day. We get too hungry between meals—then we stuff ourselves."

Karen nodded. "The lead-filled beach ball," she said, taking another sip of her coffee.

"Exactly. And that's why what we want to do is eat often, starting with breakfast, and follow all the other habits—"

"To the degree we're comfortable with them," Karen finished eagerly, setting her cup down.

Fowler nodded. "Let's go back to my car analogy. Remember that? What I want to do is change that clunker into a sports car—a sleek, healthy Ferrari! And since I have to start somewhere, the first thing I'm going to change is the gas tank. And I'm doing this to make room for that big, muscular engine that's on order. So I put in a sports-car gas tank, a much smaller tank than the one it has now. And because of the smaller tank, I have to refill it more often. So, for example, I'll eat a meal . . . "

"Breakfast."

"Breakfast. Of course. Then I'll go on a short trip, to the garden, the computer, the grocery store, then two or three hours later, when I'm starting to feel hungry, I'll eat again, *intuitively*, based solely on my body saying, Excuse me, but it's time again to refill the tank. And the food I eat can be anything—so long as it falls into the guidelines of the other habits. It can be another meal or a snack or yesterday's leftovers. Anything. And then I'm off again. On another trip, and this one will take me to noon or so, and then I'll—"

"Eat again," Karen supplied. "And again and again and again. I can do that. I *want* to do that!"

Janice cleared her throat. "Don't forget to tell her the rest."

"You tell her," Fowler said. Janice shook her head, but Fowler said to her, "You're the scientist in the family, and it's you who taught me the rest of this habit. So you tell her, because when you explained it to me, it really became the best of the best." He smiled, and then added, softly, "Please."

"Okay, okay," Janice said. She looked at Karen, cleared her throat once more, and said, "After my father began to work with the eight habits to lose weight, I realized that there was a powerful way that he could improve both his rate of weight loss and his health—"

"*Vastly* improve it," Fowler interrupted.

Janice smiled. "Yes, *vastly* improve it. And it only had to do with what he was eating, or more precisely, what he *wasn't* eating. And that was the fruits and vegetables."

Gabe threw his rings to the floor. A passing waiter picked them up and placed them on the highchair table, saying, "I have a feeling these are yours."

Janice laughed. She glanced at the waiter, and he smiled at her before walking off.

Karen, wide-eyed, looked at Janice and reached for her arm. "See! You're just another customer."

"I am, aren't I?"

Fowler beamed at her. Karen continued to smile.

Janice, whispered, "Don't do that! You're making me the center of attention! Just continue talking!" But she too was smiling.

Fowler turned to Karen, waited a moment as though trying to remember what they had been talking about, then grinned and said, "Before Janice taught me to eat fruits and vegetables, I was the proverbial meat-and-potatoes type of guy. And I still am. In fact, proud to be. But now I also keep Janice's advice about fruits and vegetables in mind, because once she explained how they work on my health, on building my powerful new Ferrari, I was amazed."

"Fruits and vegetables are really our true wonder foods," Janice said to Karen. "They're low in calories, filled with fiber, and nutrient-dense, so they give us the satisfying feeling of filling ourselves up, without that feeling of being stuffed. And because of this, every time they're a part of a meal or snack, they actually bring *down* the number of calories you eat. So you eat more bulk, feel comfortably full and satisfied, and at the same time eat fewer calories."

The server came up and refilled their coffee cups. The menus were still unopened. She said to Gabe, "What a cutie!" Then she walked away again.

Fowler said to Karen, "Fruits and vegetables *are* a true food miracle. Before Janice opened my eyes, I would eat and eat, munching on my pretzels or whatever, but I'd never feel full. Then Janice said to spice them up with a variety of vegetables or a piece of fruit, and presto, tastes better and fills me up!"

"It's their high water content," Janice said, reaching for her coffee. "That's what fruits and vegetables mostly are, water, fiber and flavor."

Fowler said to Janice, "Tell her the rest."

Janice smiled lightly. "The rest is the nutrients. Fruits and vegetables have an extraordinary amount of disease-fighting compounds in them, running the gamut from A to Z. That's why every cancer and heart organization recommends that you eat at least five servings of them a day."

"Some say nine to eleven," Fowler said, "Which is about where we are."

Janice said, "The thing that throws a lot of people off is the term *servings*. It sounds like a lot, almost like a meal by itself, but it's not."

"I used to be confused by that too," Fowler said. "Then I checked it out. Do you know that a *serving* of carrots is only 8 baby carrots? And a *serving* of grapes is only 15 grapes? I mean, I could put that away before I even realize I started eating!" He laughed. "That's why ten or so servings a day is so easy to handle . . . " Then he quickly added, "Of course I don't count servings!"

"You don't count anything, do you?" Karen said.

"Nope. Not a thing. Not when it comes to eating."

Janice said, "What the health experts who give us the number of servings we're supposed to eat *don't* say, though, is how to eat those servings in a way where it happens easily, without having to really think about it. And especially in a way that doesn't push you into that ridiculous diet mentality of feeling good or bad." She smiled. "That's where my father comes in. Those professionals may have the science down pat, but he definitely has them beaten when it comes to real life and common sense."

"Real life and common sense!" Fowler said. "My middle names." He grinned. "But really, even for a meat and potatoes guy like me, getting those servings of fruits and vegetables into my life without thinking about it is easy. In fact it's the same as when I couldn't drink all the water I wanted to, remember? I didn't want to have to work at it, put in any effort. I just wanted it to happen *automatically*. And I solved that problem with the water. Then I also solved it with the fruits and vegetables."

"*That's* why you always have them at hand," Karen said. "Your two fruit bowls, your container of cut-up veggies with dip—"

"And the vegetables with my meals, and using fruit as a dessert and a snack," Fowler continued. "What I do now, that I didn't do before Janice clued me in, is keep the thought of eating fruits and vegetables in my mind. Well, the back of my mind. So now, when I eat often, they're a *constant* part of what I eat. But now too, they're a gift, not a rule, because it's still all based on doing what I can at the moment—and then moving on with my life. No diet mentality."

"Okay." Karen said, wishing she had her notebook with her. "If I have it right, the next time I have pretzels or crackers or a bowl of cereal, or even a sandwich, I'll just include berries on the cereal or a vegetable or a fruit with the sandwich, or an apple with the pretzels. Is that it?"

"As simple as that," Fowler said. "And the combination you just listed sounds a lot like mine would be. The thing is, I don't think of it as *having* to have a fruit or vegetable anymore. I think of it as making whatever it is I'm eating more tasty and filling. I also know that not only will this wonder food melt the pounds off more quickly, it'll also give my body a regular dose of cancer-fighting and heart-disease-fighting nutrients."

Gabe began to babble. Janice leaned to him and babbled right back, getting a great toothless smile for her efforts.

Karen grinned. "Okay," she said to Fowler. "So the habit is eat often and, as much as possible, include a fruit or vegetable each time."

"Exactly. We're building our sports car from the inside out. Each time the tank gets filled, it gets filled with only the *right* amount of the *right* kind of fuel. Just the right amount and the right kind of food to get to the next fill-up. To get us from mildly hungry, to not hungry and back to mildly hungry again, as often as we need. And we do all of this within our personally tailored limits. The limits we can each live with. Sounds familiar, doesn't it?"

Karen nodded. "Sure does! The habits have to fit into my limits, my life, not the other way around."

Janice said, "Tell her how you worked with this habit when we first developed it."

"Good idea," Fowler said, "because that'll show you how our habits are built. How they form. At first I started with the premise that I'd eat a fruit or vegetable *only when it was convenient*. And that meant I was working with whatever fruit or vegetable I had on hand. And with those parameters it turned out that I was eating a fruit or vegetable two or three times a day. You know, an apple for my morning snack. Some baby carrots with lunch. Maybe something green with dinner."

"Maybe that much!" Janice said. "If the fruit wasn't cleaned or the veggies weren't prepared and waiting for you, they weren't considered convenient. I remember days when you'd eat a fruit or vegetable only once, or even not at all!"

Fowler laughed. "That's right! Convenient means convenient. Ready to eat. And that's why I started thinking about it more."

"He focused on it," Janice said, "because he wanted to make it happen without a thought."

"That's true! And when I focused on it, I realized that convenient, which for me was the key to making it simple, is really what *I* decide. What I create. And I'm also smart enough to know that with all they have going for them, once or twice a day just wasn't going to cut it. Not for me! Not for my health and weight. So just like with all the other habits, I thought it through, and in practically no time, I made *convenient* become every meal and snack. And my health took off."

Janice said, "And his pounds melted off!" She reached for her coffee.

"Then that's what I'm going to do!" Karen said. "I'm going to think about fruits and vegetables in a way I never thought of them until now—because, really, until now, I just didn't know."

Janice smiled. "You'll be amazed to know that the calorie savings you get from eating often and having a fruit and vegetable at every meal and snack, can equate to the loss of up to thirty pounds by the end of a year."

"Thirty pounds! And fight cancer and heart disease at the same time!"

Fowler grinned. "So, would you call this habit a gift?"

"A gift?" Karen said. "This is the best gift I've had in a long, long time!"

# Thirty-Three

"Okay," Fowler said, reaching for his menu. "Guess we should at least take a look. They may not mind us just gabbing and drinking coffee, but I'm getting hungry."

Janice and Karen opened their menus together.

After a couple of minutes, Fowler said to Janice, "What are you in the mood for?"

Janice shrugged. She studied the menu for another minute, then said, "Maybe pancakes. I haven't had them for a while."

Fowler turned to Karen. She was staring at the menu, expression glum. He said to her, "What are you thinking?"

Karen shook her head. "The truth is, I don't know what to choose. I mean, I don't know what would fit into the habits . . ."

Fowler grinned. "I kinda thought that was going through your mind." Looking at his own menu again, he said, "Well, the pancakes *are* a good choice if you stay away from the butter and you're careful with the syrup . . . " He continued reading the menu for a moment, then laid it flat on the table and, leaning closer to Karen, said, "Look, when we go out to eat, there are really only three things we need to be aware of. The first is the fat. These places simply don't work well with our first habit, and because of this, lots of the items on their menus are loaded with bad and ugly fats. The second thing to watch out for is the sugar—though the sugar is more easily controlled."

He flicked his menu with a finger. "And the third thing to consider is the size of the servings, because, believe it or not, the least expensive part of running a restaurant is the cost of the food itself. So they use the size of the servings as a lure to get us in."

"That's become a common practice in the industry," Janice said.

Fowler nodded. "But there are ways around each of these problems. First, there are the lower-fat items that can take the place of those that are higher in fat, like baked potatoes instead of French fries, or a fruit cup instead of hash browns. Obvious substitutions like that. And that includes the side items, like the butter they give you for your bread or the fat-filled salad dressings—those additions to the meal can easily double the amount of fat the entire meal has."

"It's still a world of choices," Karen said.

"Of course it is. It'll never be like our lowfat, personally designed haven at home, never be like my restaurant. But sensible choices can still be made."

*Why aren't there restaurants like yours?* Karen wondered. Fowler, still talking, said, "With the sugar, that's usually the dessert part of the meal, and there too the choices become obvious. Even the choice to skip the dessert and just have only a coffee. And, finally, with the size of the meal—well, the two of us can share a meal. Or order one meal and one snack, and mix and match that for two. Or ask for a doggy bag for Courage. Or, the one I usually use, just don't expect to eat it all. Know in advance that they're going to heap on the food, try to impress you that way, and just eat until you're not hungry, then ask them to take away the rest. Don't let them sucker you into lead-filled-beach-ball territory."

Karen was nodding. For another few moments she again looked at her menu, then asked Fowler, "What are you going to have?"

Fowler, looking at the menu again, tapped one of the items and said, "First, I'm going to order the fruit platter. And that'll be for all of us. We'll share it, and have it with whatever else we each order."

Janice, also looking at her menu, said, "I'll have the pancakes with one poached egg on the side."

"Good idea," Fowler said. "The egg will be your protein." Then, his eyes on the menu again, he added, "And for me, I'll have the three-egg Spanish omelet, but I'll ask them to make it with only one egg yolk, the way I do it at home, and of course that comes with the home-fried potatoes . . . " He paused for a moment, then, looking into Karen's eyes, said, "Do you remember when you ordered bacon at my house, and I told you that even though it wasn't a food I allowed into my lowfat haven, it was still available within the eight habits, because every food can be slotted into at least one of them?"

"I remember that," Karen said.

"Good. Because what I'm going to have as a side order to my omelet is an order of crispy bacon." He grinned, then, laying the menu flat on the table again, said to Karen, "Listen carefully to what I'm going to tell you next, because this is the best gift the Power of One Good Habit has to offer."

"Okay . . . " Karen said, also putting down her menu.

Fowler said, "Habit Number Eight. The last of the habits! Every once in a while, when the urge or circumstance dictates, you can knowingly, and without any sense of guilt, eat foods that don't fit into the guidelines of the other habits." He paused for a moment, letting this last habit sink in, before he said, "And this isn't just a suggestion or some sort of escape hatch or anything like that. This is a habit to be followed like all the others. To be assessed and tailored and followed. And there are valid scientific reasons for it." He looked at Janice and dipped his head.

Janice picked up the thread. "This habit is based on commonly known principles of how the body works. When your focus on all the other habits reaches a certain level, a level you'll get to quickly, what happens is that, without you realizing it, you begin to take in fewer calories than you used to."

"That's why the weight comes off," Karen said.

"Exactly," Janice said. "That's why the weight comes off. But after a while the body begins to think that this reduced number of calories is the way it's going to be from now on, so it says to itself, Well, if that's the case, if we're only going to have this number of calories from now on, then we'd better slow down our metabolism to save our fat for times of famine. But you don't want that to happen. You don't want your metabolism to slow down, because that just defeats the purpose of what you're trying to do. So you have to fool the body."

"Fool it?" Karen repeated. "What does that mean?"

"It means you have to fool it into believing that you aren't, on the whole, reducing your caloric intake. And you do that by every once in a while eating a larger-than-usual number of calories."

Fowler said to Karen, "Remember, we're not talking about pigging out here. Not talking about going back to eating the lead-filled beach ball—"

"He never does that anymore," Janice said.

"No! Never!" Fowler said. "I long ago finished with that nonsense." He smiled. "All I do to let this habit come into play is just walk away from the other habits for one meal, every once in a while. A breakfast here, a dinner there. Whatever.

"And that's a habit?" Karen said. "I mean, eating foods that don't fit into the other habits is a habit? It's something I'm supposed to do?"

"That's right. Eating foods that don't fit into the other habits, every once in a while, when the urge or the circumstances dictate, is one of the habits. The last of the eight habits. It's something you're supposed to do. *Have* to do! And, just like with all the other habits, there's no specific timing to it, no numbers to count, very little to think about."

"And no guilt? You said that, didn't you? No guilt."

Janice laughed. "At the beginning, that was *his* biggest problem too," she said, pointing at her father. "Feeling guilty about going off the other habits, having something that the other habits said to bypass. And he didn't want to do it. Even though he understood the science and explained it to me, he didn't want to do it."

"But I did do it," Fowler said. "At the occasional meal I simply ate a *little* more than I usually would, or I ate something that didn't fit into my lowfat and low-sugar haven at home. Because I wanted to see what would happen. And it works! That blip, that jolt to the system, keeps the body off-guard, keeps it thinking that everything is the way it used to be. This habit doesn't make you put on weight, because it keeps your metabolism up, and that keeps pushing your weight down." He smiled at the expression of dubious glee on Karen's face.

Janice said, "This habit also clearly shows that the Power of One Good Habit isn't a diet. It's not something you start and eventually stop. What it is, as my father keeps saying, is a way to incrementally, and consistently, over your lifetime, gain health through an understanding of moderation and good nutritional practices. You're gaining health and losing weight by understanding how to defeat those cultural forces that are making fortunes seducing people into buying what they have to offer."

"With this habit," Fowler said, "though we're fighting a war—and it *is* a war—the Power of One Good Habit always remains partnered with the real world. And in the real world, there are situations that come up when following the other habits is just not possible. That's when *I* let this last habit come into play. When some editor invites me to dinner or when a publisher puts out a spread for an office party, or for any holiday. Or," Fowler said, looking directly into Karen's eyes, "simply when I get the urge to have something I haven't had in a while, like bacon."

Karen said, "You once told me there was a way I could eat my ice cream and savor it, without feeling guilty . . . "

"You remembered that?"

"How could I forget?"

"Well, this is how," Fowler said. "With this last habit."

Karen smiled. She shook her head in wonder.

"So," Fowler continued, "leaving the other habits once in a while isn't only one of the habits, it's also an important part of the whole process. First, it works on the metabolism, keeps that running at the speed it should. And second, it forces the habits to fit into the real world, because it says that any food eaten once in a while—even foods that don't fit into the other habits—are acceptable. And that means that in the big picture, the real-life picture, any and every food is okay. There are absolutely no exceptions to this habit. The type of food just doesn't matter."

For a moment no one spoke. Then Karen said, "The eight habits do fit *everyone*, don't they? They fit all of us like a second skin. And they're made to wear for the rest of our lives."

"You got it!" Fowler said. For a moment he remained quiet, then, looking into Karen's eyes, he added, "Now you know all eight habits. So the thing to do is review them. Understand them. Let them work their way through your mind. Then, when you're ready, begin each one—slowly—continually adjusting it to fit you and the particular moment. And remember, let each habit be result-driven. Let your depth of focus for each one grow with the excitement those results create. That'll drive the whole process. And at the same time know that once the eight habits are inside you, the tools to control your nutritional health and weight are in your hands. And also know that you're living in the real world, in real time, with real circumstances and urges and walls, and that they're all a part of the whole. All accounted for."

"It has to work," Karen said with certainty.

"Once you have the knowledge," Fowler said, "you can decide to ignore that knowledge, pretend you're still blind to the battle going on around you, pretend you don't know the effect the enemy is having on your health and your family's health—"

"That's when you become your *own* enemy," Karen said.

"Yes. If you ignore what you now know, and go on the way you used to, you become your own enemy, with no one to blame for the negative results but yourself. But if you do accept the knowledge; if you accept, at any time, any part of any of the eight habits, then the power is in your hands, and you can't fail."

Janice said, "It's *never* an all or nothing situation. You use what you need of the habits—a bit of this one, a bit of that—depending on the circumstances at hand."

"That's right," Fowler said. "Always remember, you're not *attempting* something, so you can't fail at it. You're doing it! You're taking a step, then another, and another, toward better health. And each of those steps is a success in itself! And each success adds to the next, building greater and greater successes. And if a wall gets in your way, and it *will*! Then you take it down when you can, and continue on."

For a moment they sat without speaking, then Fowler said, "Okay! Time to eat!" He signaled the server. She came over, lifted her pad from her waistband, and said, "You folks ready to order?"

"Yes," Fowler answered. "And thank you for your patience." He looked at the menu again, but before pointing out what he wanted, he turned to the server once more and said, "The first thing I'm going to need is water. Water with lemon. A tall glass of cold water with a slice of lemon." He grinned at Karen and Janice, then to the server, added, "You'd better make that three."

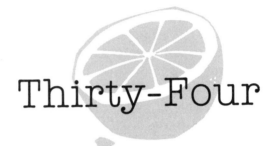

# Thirty-Four

Karen sat on the living room couch, holding Gabe, and waited for Gary to come home. She kept saying to herself, *You can do this. You have to do this. You have to find the courage!*

Gabe, cranky all afternoon, still wavered between tears and a heavy, toothless pout. Karen lifted him close to her lips and, wishing he could understand, whispered, "No matter what happens, I don't want you to worry, because it's going to be okay."

Just then Gary opened the front door and stepped into the townhouse. In a single movement, he shucked his jacket onto the hall bench and turned toward the living room.

Karen said, "Gary."

"What?" Gary answered, walking into the room. He took a seat on the easy chair and reached for the TV remote.

"We have to talk," Karen said.

For an instant Gary looked at her, lips tightly sealed, then he turned back to the television and clicked it on.

"We can't go on like this," Karen continued.

In a blunt, dismissive tone, Gary said, "I'm hungry."

Karen closed her eyes, slowly shook her head. For the moment Gabe remained quiet.

"Are you deaf?" Gary said. "I just came in and I'm hungry."

"No," Karen answered, lifting her eyes to his.

"No? What do you mean, no?"

"I mean we can't go on like this."

Gary stared at her.

"Gary," Karen said, "it doesn't have to be this way, with this much anger. We were good together once. Don't you remember? We fought. But then we made up. We laughed together. We were there for each other."

For a long moment, Gary said nothing.

Karen said, "Gary."

"Things change," Gary said, still not looking at her.

"But they can change back," Karen replied quickly. "If we try, I mean *really* try. If we *both* try hard, and if we remember how it used to be." She leaned forward. "Please, Gary. We can do it! We can get help. Go for counseling . . . "

Karen watched Gary's jaws tighten, his muscles stiffen. She watched him turn back to the television and say once again, "I'm hungry."

Karen's own expression grew determined. She took a deep breath, stood up and, holding securely to Gabe, said, "Then I've had enough, Gary. I'm a person too. I'm not your doormat, I'm not the maid, and I'm not someone who lives here but sleeps on the couch. I won't live this way any more. I want you out."

"What?"

"I said I want you out!" Karen yelled. "Get out of this house! I won't live like this anymore. I'm tired of the insults, of trying to keep you happy, of being a failure just because you say I'm a failure!"

Gabe started to cry. Karen began to rock him, trying to be as comforting as possible.

Gary's expression hadn't changed. "If you're finished, I'm still hungry."

"Didn't you hear what I said?"

Gary shrugged, the movement slow, filled with disdain. Then he suddenly shouted, "The show's over, Karen! You made your splash and you're not going anywhere! If you don't want to sleep on the couch, then don't! I don't care. Is that what you wanted to hear?"

After a long pause, Karen whispered, "Yes." Then, shaking her head, she added, "But it's not enough. I need more than that." She brought her head close to Gabe's, kissing his tears.

Gary, turning back to the TV, said, "What more? What do you mean, more?"

"More, Gary. I need more than just permission to sleep in my own bed. I need respect."

"Then respect yourself," Gary said without looking at her.

For a moment, Karen was silent. Then she said, "I do respect myself. I'm learning how to do that."

"Well, good for you."

"And I want you to leave."

"Why do you keep saying that?" Gary yelled, snapping his head toward Karen again. "That's not what you want. You and the kid can't manage on your own, you know that! Not the way you are!"

"I want you to leave."

Gary turned back to the TV.

Again Karen said, "I want you to leave."

Gary remained silent, making no movement, his eyes still glued to the screen.

Karen stepped around to the front of the easy chair. She looked down at Gary and felt, for the first time in her married life, that he was afraid to look at her. Afraid to lift his head, to see what was in her eyes. She said, very quietly now, "Gary, I've thought this through, and I've made my decision. I won't continue living this way. My life is important too.

228

And now I want you to leave. If you want, you can go for help, talk to someone about your anger. And then we'll see. And if you don't, that'll be your choice. But now, I want you to leave." With this she turned from him and stepped to the window, repeating, "Go, Gary. I don't need you anymore."

For a long moment there was no sound between them. Then Gary said, "Karen."

But she didn't turn to him. For an instant she felt guilt, wavered with that, then fear that he'd get violent, storm from the chair and grab her. Then she returned to her original sense of determination, and let that quality shunt the other feelings aside, bolster her newfound strength, her growing confidence. She forced herself to keep her back to Gary even when he yelled, "You're going to regret this, Karen. Mark my words!"

She remained steadfast while he stormed to the door and slammed it shut behind him, then watched as he hurried to his car and, with a squeal of tires, drove off.

Now, she knew, it was just her and Gabe.

She brought her head down to Gabe's, touched his cheek with hers, felt fresh tears rise to just below the surface, and told herself, *No! There are a million good reasons to cry. But Gary isn't one of them. Not any more.*

She was scared. She admitted it to herself. *Take one step,* she thought, *then another. Remember that each step is a success in itself. Concentrate on that. Only think about that.* She took a deep breath, then whispered to Gabe, "I did it, didn't I? I came up to the wall and went through it. I went through it. I was scared and I faced it and went through it!" She smiled, feeling relief, feeling . . . hungry.

She went into the kitchen and put Gabe into the highchair.

All she'd had to eat today was breakfast with Fowler and Janice, then a grilled chicken sandwich and a pear for lunch. She'd eaten lunch at the park, sitting on a bench, while Gabe ate his in the stroller. Then she'd circled the park twice, needing the fresh air in her lungs and the feeling that she was moving her body. The rest of the afternoon was spent thinking about what she was going to do when Gary got home, building up the courage to go through with it.

Almost without thought, she opened the freezer door and reached for the ice cream, reached for an old friend. Then she thought, *No.* She had another idea, a better one. She let the door close.

She was smiling, beginning to feel the excitement and importance of what she'd done. "I did it! I took down my wall!" She laughed, then found herself crying. *But they're good tears,* she thought. *From now on, my life is going to be different. I made a choice. I gave Gary the option to do the same thing. I'll try again, if he wants to, but there has to be an effort on his part. I've taken a tremendous step forward and I'm not going back!*

*The Power of One Good Habit is in me now! I learned the last of the eight habits today. That knowledge is mine now, and it can't be erased.*

*Courage,* she thought. *Creativity. Tailor the eight habits to the moment. Take a step, one small step, then another, knowing that each step is a success in itself. Begin a constant, incremental movement toward better health and toward a better tomorrow.*

She opened the fridge door this time. She took out a lemon, cut a slice from it, then dropped the slice into a glass and filled it with water.

#  Thirty-Five

Fowler had Gabe in his arms when he opened the front door. Gabe squealed in delight as he recognized his mother. Karen reached for him, saying, "Hi, there! Did you miss me? I hope you were a good boy!"

Janice, right behind Fowler, said, "How did it go?"

Karen smiled. She was wearing a stylish suit with matching shoes, and in the past seven months had lost twenty-six pounds. The weight loss showed on her face and on her body and in her spirit.

Fowler had told her to go slowly and experiment with the habits. "Make them really yours," he'd said, "not carbon copies of mine. Work at having the eight habits, one by one, become invisible in your life."

And that was what Karen did. She relished her steady gain in health, knowing that her steady decline in weight was permanent. She knew that every pound lost was not the result of dieting, but of continuously incorporating small, lasting changes into her nutritional lifestyle, her nutritional mind-set.

She'd had fits and starts, especially during the first few months while she and Gary struggled with the difficult, initial steps she knew were needed if their marriage was going to work. Gary had at first refused, then agreed to getting help with his anger. And in the past two weeks, at Gary's request, they had progressed to counseling as a couple.

"I'm hopeful," Karen had told Janice. "I know there's a good man in there, because that's who I married. And he's a terrific father; that's more apparent every day. But I'm also realistic. Making a relationship work requires effort. It doesn't just happen on its own."

She had accepted and even anticipated those initial fits and starts with the eight habits. And she knew too that walls were also going to show themselves—they already had. But through it all she had never let herself get caught up in the diet mentality of anxiety and guilt.

She had read and reread her notes, finding more in them each time, until each of the habits became firmly planted in her mind. Then, gradually, with one small step after another, the Power of One Good Habit became a part of her life.

Only this morning, when she'd had coffee with Janice and Fowler before leaving Gabe with them, she had likened the eight habits to friends. "When you first meet someone," she said, "it takes time for that person to become a friend, and then a good friend, and then the best of friends. You have to get to know them first, understand them, accept and trust them. And that's the way I approached each of the eight habits, anticipating the best, but taking the time I needed."

Now she said to Janice and Fowler, "I got it! I got the loan!"

"Yes!" Janice shouted, pumping a fist in the air.

"Well, what do you know," Fowler said. "I didn't think they'd be that smart."

"They loved the idea!" Karen said. "Especially how I'm going to team up with my boss to showcase his restaurant equipment. The bank manager himself said I could count on him becoming a faithful customer." She laughed. "I can hardly wait to tell Sue and the others in my office. Most of them are already working with the habits, my boss and his wife included! And now they're getting their families and friends involved too. Even the people who don't need to lose weight are excited about it, about having a way to get a handle on their health. That's one of the reasons I want this restaurant, so it can become a meeting place for those who want to learn about the Power of One Good Habit, who want to lose weight without dieting." She shook her head as though in wonder, then said, "It'll be small, but perfect! And mine! And there'll be no shortcuts taken. Everything I've learned and every ounce of my courage and creativity will go into it."

"You told him about the menu?" Fowler prodded her. "How each item will have the recipe printed too, so your customers can try it for themselves at home? Adapt it to their own habits, let it become a new comfort food?"

"Yes. He was so impressed with that."

"And the takeout counter," Janice said. "That it'll be called the Energy Bank. You told him about that?"

Karen, smiling broadly, nodded.

"What about the name?" Fowler wanted to know.

"With your permission," Karen said, "I'd like to call it The Power of One Good Habit."

Fowler nodded. Karen could see him swallow hard. Then he said, "I would be thrilled for you to use that name. I never imagined anyone else would appreciate it, understand how much significance it has."

"Thank you," Karen said softly. Then, excited again, she added, "The Power of One Good Habit, a restaurant based on nutritional sanity. And it'll be innovative. I want to give demonstrations of how to find and eliminate fat and sugar, how to work with the other habits. I'm going to start clubs— Power of One Good Habit clubs! So families and groups of friends can get together, become involved and help each other take control of their health and weight."

"It's what we've needed for a long time now," Fowler said. Then he turned to Janice. "Looks like this is a day for good news." He stepped closer to her and put a hand on her shoulder.

"I accepted a job offer this morning," Janice told Karen. "They called just after you left."

For a moment Karen had no words, then she rushed over to Janice and, with Gabe still in her arms, leaned down and hugged her. "I'm so happy for you!"

Janice said, "It's a little scary. But I'm excited. Most of it will be over the Internet. But there will be some meetings. I'll have to get on a plane and fly to conferences. I've never even been on a plane before."

Fowler beamed.

Karen said, "The Power of One Good Habit got you this far, and from here it will take you to wherever you want to go. You, Fowler, me—and the world!"

*When it comes to losing weight*
*and gaining health,*
*anything that doesn't sound like*
*good common sense,*
*anything that isn't simple sense,*
*is usually nonsense.*

―

# What Now?

Now that you've read the DIET FREE novel, *Water with Lemon* and experienced each character's difficulties, triumphs and ultimate transformation, what are *you* going to do next?

You began by following Karen as she learned what the habits were, then watched while she carefully thought through each habit and saw how it could work for *her* and fit into *her* own particular lifestyle.

**Like Karen, are *you* now ready to fully embrace these eight habits? Will you allow them to become a constant and invisible force in your life?**

## Turn *Knowing* into *Doing*

We know how hard it is to turn *knowing* into *doing*. And we know that even after reading this eye-opening book, you probably need more guidance, education and tools to sustain you on your DIET FREE journey. Zonya has the answers, guides and tools to help you take the DIET FREE habits to the next level with the **DIET FREE Lifestyle Program.**

- This complete program will give you even more inspiration and education with weekly video and audio seminars on each of the habits—all delivered in Zonya's entertaining style.

- You will become more empowered for finding ways to adopt the eight habits into your life with the complete *DIET FREE Lifestyle Guide*. This robust book is full of commonsense action tips, valuable reference charts, habit homework assignments and a focused eight-point plan for exercise—one to go along with each habit you are learning.

- The "Everyday Fitness: Movement Training Program" workout DVD will help you abandon pain, strengthen your core and gain the flexibility you need to make exercise become as much a part of who you are as your own middle name.

- Using the pocket-sized *DIET FREE Habit Tracker,* you'll be able to record and witness the daily, weekly and monthly changes in your health as you incorporate all of the eight habits and find what works for you in *real* life for the *rest* of your life.

- And having the support of the DIET FREE Lifestyle program, you'll be inspired to start cleaning out your refrigerator and cupboards and making a fresh start, just like Karen did. On your journey to optimum health, you'll acquire new comfort foods, discover healthy recipes and shop differently with the help of Zonya's *Lickety-Split Meals for Health Conscious People on the Go!* cookbook.


**Watch video highlights of the program and learn more at www.DIETFREE.com**

# A Word About
# Exercise

As professionals certified in health and fitness, we cannot let you put down this book without a special note about exercise. Exercise played a vital role in Karen's weight-loss success and overall improved health. And we realize that it is just as difficult to turn knowing into doing when it comes to good exercise habits as it is for developing good eating habits. Therefore, we have made the conscious decision not to address exercise at length in this book. The habits around building an active lifestyle are too important to simply tack onto a book already filled with healthy habits about nutrition.

The benefits of exercise far exceed boosting your metabolism and burning fat. Aerobic activities improve your immune system while fighting heart disease, type 2 diabetes, cancer, dementia and depression. Adding strength-training bumps up these benefits even more by helping you maintain proper strength and balance, and helps prevent insulin resistance and osteoporosis.

When you commit to be fit, are curious and courageous enough to discover your "fitness love" and surround yourself with like-minded friends, then exercise will become top-of-mind and define who you are as much as your own middle name! When you think of exercise as something you "get" to do instead of something you "have" to do, your life will truly change forever.

You'll find that exercise gets the full airing it deserves in the complete DIET FREE Lifestyle Program. This program coaches you through the eight DIET FREE habits you just learned with Karen, plus our eight-point plan for exercise. We call it, **"Every day exercise . . . and make it your middle name."**

**Visit www.DIETFREE.com
to learn more.**

# The Eight DIET FREE Habits
# That Will Change Your Life!

Just as Karen learned, these seemingly simple habits when adopted one after the other—at a pace that works for you—will become the invisible force that changes your life. After reading this book, you'll realize that it's not *just* the habits, but the way they're presented in this story that makes DIET FREE weight loss so absolutely doable! Get ready to ditch the diet mentality and enjoy living DIET FREE forever!

—Zonya and Stephen

**D**rink water . . . and think before you drink anything else.

Water is the body's most important nutrient. It provides the healthy internal "car wash" you need for better concentration, fighting diseases and flushing away fat. Begin drinking water first thing each morning and add lemon or lime for a refreshing taste change throughout the day. Replace calorie-filled sodas with water because unconsciously drinking high-sugar beverages can account for up to 50 extra pounds you may be carrying around. And drinking just one can of soda per day can double your chances of type 2 diabetes.

**I**nclude breakfast . . . and stop eating two to three hours before bedtime.

People who include breakfast eat fewer calories daily than people who don't. And when you stop "unconscious" evening snacking, you'll save another 300 or more calories daily and be ready to start the next day right by eating a nutritious breakfast. This habit won't make you weigh less after just one day or even a week. But after a full year of including breakfast and eliminating evening snacking, you could be 30 to 50 pounds lighter!

# E at often . . . and include a fruit or vegetable each time.

Eating often keeps your hunger hormones under control and prevents you from feeling starved and then overeating. By including a fruit or vegetable with every meal or snack, you'll be satisfied with fewer calories while loading up on disease-fighting, fat-flushing vitamins, minerals and antioxidants. This 200–300 daily calorie savings may not seem like much, but this habit alone can melt off 20 to 30 pounds in a year while protecting you from heart disease, type 2 diabetes and cancer.

# T ame your sweet tooth . . . and naturally eat as little sugar as possible.

First, put a halt to your sweet cravings by eating fruit. Fruit is nature's candy and a natural way to give your brain the simple carbohydrates it needs to prevent sweet cravings. Then, learn to dial down the level of sweetness you desire by gradually choosing cereals that are lower in sugar, unsweetened beverages and desserts made with half the typical sugar. Finally, learn to recognize what is "sweet" and plan to enjoy two small sweet treats a day. Once your taste buds no longer enjoy an intensely sweet taste, you'll naturally eat less sugar without feeling deprived. Adopting this habit will save you 100–500 calories a day, helping you to lose 10–50 pounds by the end of one year!

# Find the fat . . . and know the good, the bad and the ugly.

Choose foods that are as low in fat as possible, then add back limited amounts of good fat. Become a no-fried-foods person and begin exploring low-fat cooking methods. Choose lean meats, low-fat cheeses and skim milk. Clear your pantry of anything labeled "partially hydrogenated" or "hydrogenated." Then add back limited portions of unsaturated and omega 3 good fats, the kind found in nuts, seeds, olive oil and salmon. This is the easiest way to eliminate the bad saturated and ugly trans fats while getting just enough of the good unsaturated and omega 3 fats your body needs. Not only will this habit help you lose weight by reducing the total amount of fat you eat, it will also help you stay on the safe side of the statistic that one out of every two people dies of heart disease.

# Replace processed food with wholesome . . . and shop natural, close-to-the-farm.

Choose whole-grain bread, rice and pasta instead of white. Go for fresh meat and cheese, not processed. And don't be suckered into thinking fruit-flavored snacks or vegetable chips are healthy alternatives to real fruit and vegetables. Wholesome food has less sugar, fat, sodium and chemicals and provides more fiber and natural nutrients. Natural, close-to-the-farm food also helps normalize blood sugar and blood pressure, while providing greater hunger control than processed and chemically enhanced food.

**E**at until no longer hungry . . . and stop the lead-filled beach ball!

This is the most difficult habit to master but the most important to adopt. Share an entrée, quit the "clean-plate club," eat slowly and savor every bite. Learn to enjoy feeling light on your feet instead of stuffed, like a lead-filled beach ball. When you regularly stop eating when you're beginning to feel no longer hungry, you can save as many as 400 calories a day. That equates to 40 pounds lost in a year's time. Combine that with ending *emotional* (mindless) eating, and you could drop another 20 pounds. Now you've lost 60 pounds in a year from adopting just this one habit alone!

**E**very once in awhile, when the urge or circumstance dictates, it's all right to live outside the guidelines of the other habits.

And understand that this habit is just as important as the others. All the other habits are designed to make your body lose weight, and when that happens, your body compensates by slowing down your metabolism. To keep your metabolism stoked and burning calories at the appropriate rate, this habit tells your body there's no need to store calories because there's no pending famine. This habit makes the other habits fit into your life and eliminates the diet mentality of feeling deprived and guilty. And that's because this isn't a diet—this is living!

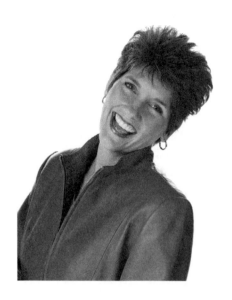

# America's
# Nutrition Leader

## Zonya Foco,
### RD, CHFI, CSP

Zonya is on a mission to win the war on obesity, diabetes and heart disease. Her easy humor and dynamic style drive home the message that when it comes to health and nutrition, each of us can change our lives with **The Power of One Good Habit**. As a teen who saw her own weight bounce up and down, ending each diet at a higher number on the scale, Zonya is now motivating people everywhere with a common-sense approach to healthy eating through her TV show, "Zonya's Health Bites," her popular cookbook, *Lickety-Split Meals for Health Conscious People on the Go*, and the DIET FREE novel, *Water with Lemon*.

Before launching her speaking and writing career in 1994, Zonya received her Bachelor of Science degree in dietetics and worked for eight years as a clinical nutritionist for the Michigan Heart and Vascular Institute at St. Joseph Mercy Hospital in Ann Arbor. Through her experience with these clients, Zonya discovered that simple core habits are the secret to lifelong health and good nutrition.

The only Registered Dietitian (RD) and Certified Health and Fitness Instructor (CHFI) in the country to have earned the prestigious Certified Speaking Professional (CSP) designation, Zonya's boundless energy inspires audiences across North America to stop dieting and start living the healthy life they deserve.

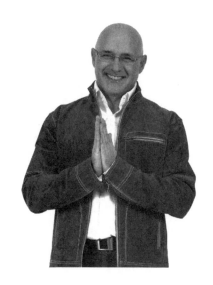

# America's Health Novelist

## Stephen Moss,
### CFT, LWMC

He knew there had to be a better way. And he found it!

Stephen grew up in a household where being overweight was the norm. But when his own genetics kicked into the overweight gear, he decided to fight back. That's when he discovered that the world of weight-loss information was a mix of mind-boggling jargon and unnecessarily complex science. It was difficult and dull and often led nowhere.

He found a path through the maze and went on to bring his weight under control, becoming along the way a Certified Fitness Trainer (CFT) and Lifestyle and Weight Management Consultant (LWMC). A lifelong passion for fitness and weight control had begun.

But Stephen had another passion—writing novels—and he realized that his newfound knowledge put him in a unique position. He created the characters he would need to tell the story and joined forces with Zonya Foco, RD. Together they deliver the true answer to weight loss and healthy eating in the first-ever health novel, *Water with Lemon*.

Thanks to Stephen, a new genre is born, and the world of weight management will never be the same!